Beyond CAHPS

A Guide for Achieving Patient- and Family-Centered Care

Janiece Gray, MHA, BSW, CPXP

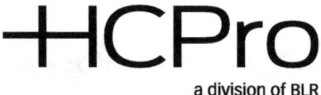

Beyond CAHPS: A Guide for Achieving Patient- and Family-Centered Care is published by HCPro, a division of BLR.

Copyright © 2016 HCPro, a division of BLR

All rights reserved. Printed in the United States of America.   5 4 3 2 1

Download the additional materials of this book at *www.hcpro.com/downloads/12531*

ISBN: 978-1-68308-120-3

No part of this publication may be reproduced, in any form or by any means, without prior written consent of HCPro or the Copyright Clearance Center (978-750-8400). Please notify us immediately if you have received an unauthorized copy.

HCPro provides information resources for the healthcare industry.

HCPro is not affiliated in any way with The Joint Commission, which owns the JCAHO and Joint Commission trademarks.

Janiece Gray, MHA, BSW, CPXP, Author

Jay Kumar, Associate Product Manager

Erin Callahan, Vice President, Product Development & Content Strategy

Elizabeth Petersen, Executive Vice President, Healthcare

Matt Sharpe, Production Supervisor

Vincent Skyers, Design Services Director

Vicki McMahan, Sr. Graphic Designer/Layout

Jason Gregory, Cover Designer

Advice given is general. Readers should consult professional counsel for specific legal, ethical, or clinical questions.

Arrangements can be made for quantity discounts. For more information, contact:

HCPro

100 Winners Circle, Suite 300

Brentwood, TN 37027

Telephone: 800-650-6787 or 781-639-1872

Fax: 800-785-9212

Email: *customerservice@hcpro.com*

Visit HCPro online at *www.hcpro.com* and *www.hcmarketplace.com*

Contents

Dedication vii

About the Author ix

Preface xi

Section 1: Introduction 1

Chapter 1: Moving Beyond the Compulsories 3
Definitions 5

Chapter 2: CAHPS = Compulsories—Necessary But Insufficient . . 13
Tip of the Iceberg 15

Chapter 3: Connection to the WIIFMs—Reasons to Care 19
What If It Were Me or My Family?: Putting Yourself in the Patient's Shoes . 20
Employee Engagement and Physician Satisfaction 22
The Financial Component 23
Public Image and Transparency 25
Connection Between Patient Experience and Patient Engagement 28

Section 2: Foundation/Connection and Collaboration—Patients and People 31

Contents

Chapter 4: Patients Are the Reason We Exist 33
Patient and Family Advisory Councils 35

Chapter 5: People Are the Reason We Excel 61
Connection Between Employee Engagement and Patient Experience . . .63
Connecting People to Purpose 66
Active Listening 67
Frontline Example 68
An Engaged Culture…You Can Feel It 69
Building a Culture. 70

Section 3: Structure. 75

Chapter 6: Setting Up for Success 77
Scope 78
Setting Up for Success: Do You Need a CXO? .79
Internal Support Structure 81
Executive Sponsorship 88
What to Look For in a Patient Experience Leader 92

Section 4: Data 101

Chapter 7: Sources of Data and Supporting Technology 103
Types of Measures 104
Survey Partner 105
The Grass is Always Greener 106
Supplement to Aid in Improvement. 107
Augment With Appropriate Technology to Inform 108
Rounding Tools. 109
The Electronic Medical Record 113

Chapter 8: The Display and Use of Data 115
Percentiles 118
Better Comparisons 119
Composites 124
Transparency. 125
Enterprise Data Warehouse 127

Section 5: Methods 131

Chapter 9: Communication Counts 133
Key Care Practices Across the Continuum..........................134
At the Heart of It All: Empathy...................................136
Three Good Things 142
Mindfulness 145

Chapter 10: Spectrum of Strategies 151
Key Strategies for Improvement 153
Get Creative 155
Black Box CME™ 155
Simulation: Act Your Way Into a New Way of Being 158
No Silver Bullet, But ... .168

Chapter 11: Traversing the Trajectory—The Journey to Improvement 179
You're on the Journey, Now What?..............................182

Chapter 12: Case Study: Allina Health.................... 187
Organizational Background 187
Historical Context...187
Current and Recent Activity 189
Patient and Family Partnership Program 191
Data 195
Bedside Shift Handover 199
Results 204
Lessons Learned..205
Where is Allina Health Headed? 208

Chapter 13: Case Study: El Camino Hospital 211
Historical Context...211
Lessons Learned..217
What's Next? 220

Chapter 14: Conclusion 221

Dedication

For Betty, who told me to "Go downstairs and write" and encouraged me throughout!

About the Author

Janiece Gray, MHA, BSW, CPXP, is a gifted communicator and consultant who is passionate about improving care by helping caregivers and healthcare professionals do a better job of understanding, connecting and engaging with patients. She is a cofounder and CEO of DTA Associates Inc., a healthcare consulting firm focused on helping providers achieve patient-centered improvement goals. Janiece and her team are uniquely positioned to partner with clinical care teams and operations leadership to develop custom solutions to enhance patient experience, improve clinical outcomes, and streamline processes. Janiece has more than 20 years of experience in patient care, healthcare administration and operations, performance improvement, and patient experience. She earned a bachelor's of science in social work from Bethel University and a master's in healthcare administration from the University of Minnesota. Janiece worked in a variety of progressive leadership roles at Allina Health in Minneapolis, developing new prevention programs as well as new care environments. Using her Lean training and her Black Belt in Six Sigma, she has developed and led service and performance improvement training programs to create more efficiencies and opportunities for better patient care. Additionally, Janiece has not only led performance improvement and patient experience departments but has also developed and leads empathy, patient experience, and quality improvement training programs. She loves to shadow and coach physicians and other care team members on ways they can enhance their patient communication.

Preface

One of my earliest memories was when I was 3 years old and my mom and her friend and I went to the mall in Harrisburg, Pennsylvania. We spent the evening shopping, and as we went back to our car (a light blue Ford Pinto) at the end of the night, my mom's friend, Cheryl, looked at my mom and asked, "Does she *always* talk this much?" My mom politely smiled and nodded. Later that evening back at our house, I looked at my mom and said, "I know I talk a lot … it's just because I have so much to say!"

I love that story because it's very true of me, even today. When I was asked to write a book about one of my passions—patient experience and patient- and family-centered care—I couldn't believe it! Not only was it a dream come true, but as always, I realized I had so much to say.

When I was in junior high, they had us do one of those career exploration exercises to help us figure out what we wanted to be when we grew up. For a while I wanted to be an interior designer, then a financial planner. But somehow I never really had a clear vision for what I wanted to be when I grew up. Now, as an adult, I realize it's because many of the jobs I've held and careers I've been fortunate enough to be in didn't exist back then. Almost every position I've been in has been a newly created one for the organization: social worker and outreach coordinator for a Parkinson's specialty clinic and nonprofit fundraising association; wellness intern focused on building a medical fitness center for a large senior housing company; director of operations

Preface

who designed and built a medical specialty center with clinics, lab, radiology, and a surgery center; performance improvement consultant within a newly formed Lean/Six Sigma division for a healthcare organization; director of patient experience for systemwide improvements; founding partner of a consulting firm; and leader of a patient experience practice.

There's a theme there, and it made me realize that so many of us are in jobs and roles that didn't exist 15, 10, or even five years ago. When I first took on my role leading patient experience at Allina Health, it wasn't as popular as it is now. My resources for improvement and mentoring were not as robust as they are today. However, I am so fortunate for the many people and connections that helped to teach me what I was able to learn and lead. I'm unbelievably grateful to Carrie Brady, Esther Burlingame, Lynn Ehrmantraut, Colleen Feldhausen, David Medvedeff, and Dale Shaller for their friendship and leadership.

In addition to those connections and influences, there were so many amazing leaders and partners from within Allina, as well as other organizations, that helped to shape my experiences and helped form the basis for writing this book.

People like Dr. Tierza Stephan, Dr. Ben Bache-Wiig, Dr. Penny Wheeler, Dr. Steve Bergeson, Mary Jo Morrison, Tomi Ryba, Cheryl Reinking, RJ Salus, Tracy Laibson, Janet Wied, Amy Edwards, Jay Scott, Mike Wenzel, Tracy Kirby, Gretchen Leiterman, Richelle Jader, and Dr. Kurt Isenberger. I specifically want to highlight and thank contributing chapter authors Dr. Steve Bergeson, Tracy Laibson, Janet Wied, and RJ Salus, for the case studies that they took the time to write for me. I'm grateful for my partner Kevin Campbell, who not only authored several chapters but also proved to be an excellent editor and cheerleader for me in this process. I also want to thank those who graciously gave their time and shared their expertise to help research and fine-tune various aspects of this work: Lynn Ehrmantraut, Leslie Balbecki, Mike Wenzel, Jay Scott, Dr. Tierza Stephan, Nicole Braegelmann, and Jennifer Schugel. There are a few others whose voices have impacted me as their words echoed in my writing—thanks to Doug Pagitt, Mark Dixon, and Jessica Anderson. And last but not least, thanks to my husband Jason and our three little ones who challenge, inspire, and support—Emma, Alyson, and Avery.

Since leaving Allina, I've had the privilege of working with several organizations helping and assisting them in their journey to improvement in striving for patient- and family-centered care and patient experience. What I've learned with them, building off of my journey at Allina, is that A) there's so much to do in this space; B) anything is possible; and C) it's always more of a journey than a destination. In some ways, that's great job security for those working in this field.

And yet, there are frustrations. I'd be remiss if I didn't admit that this is some of the more challenging work that I have ever encountered. This work is very personal, and so often the people that we're trying to influence can be defensive. The data and measurement for outcomes are tricky at times and often directional at best. There's a significant lag in the measurement between performance improvement activities and actual results. And there's increasing pressure from the payment system and organizational leaders to go further, farther, faster.

That being said, this is truly some of the most rewarding work I've ever been a part of, and I truly feel that in this place, I've found my passion. My hope is that, by sharing some of the experiences, lessons learned, and ideas about how to avoid many of the potholes I've fallen into and helped others get out of, you too can experience greater success on your journey.

Section 1

Introduction

Chapter 1

Moving Beyond the Compulsories

My first introduction to work in quality and performance improvement was at Allina Health under the direction of then–Chief Clinical Officer (CCO) Penny Wheeler, MD. As Penny assumed the CCO role, she had an approach to and a platform for her vision for quality deemed the 4 C's: compulsories, connection, collaboration, and community. While it sounds like a simple model, realizing this to its fullest is both daunting and inspiring. Little did I know at the time, this model would become the basis of my approach not only to quality and performance improvement but also to patient experience, and ultimately to patient- and family-centered care.

Let's look a little deeper at this approach:

- Compulsories

    Any time you're working in an area with tons of rules and regulations, it's easy to get bogged down in the "must do's," the "cans," and the "cannots" of the work. These are the compulsories. Many people get lost and stuck in this place and focus only on the letter of the law, whether we are hitting the measure, and the resulting color on the scorecard. These are things we must do (hence "compulsories"); however, when you're trying to engage care team members about quality, focusing solely on the compulsories is not what will ultimately motivate them.

- Connection

    To look beyond the minimum requirements and regulations and to consider how we can make a difference and improve takes connection: connection with caregivers and the care team members providing the care, as well as with the patients and family members receiving the care. This means leaving our offices or cubicle land and getting out—to the sites, to the units, to the people, to the physicians, to the patients—and connecting with them about what is meaningful to them with regard to whatever quality metric is being considered.

- Collaboration

    Making lasting changes and sustaining true process improvement is rarely achieved in silos. Whether within units or between sites within a larger organization, breaking down those silos and finding ways to collaborate and learn from one another is the key to success. Systemic change can only occur when we work together to understand why some areas can achieve success while others struggle, and when we creatively problem solve together.

- Community

    Historically in healthcare, we've been pretty siloed and myopic to only think about what goes on within the walls of *our* organization. This wasn't selfishly derived so much as it was congruent with how we were paid. In a fee-for-service world, we competed on volumes with our rival health systems and were paid accordingly. With the shift to value-based payments and ultimately to accountability for an entire population, it's no longer enough to think only within our organizations. To truly achieve this requires partnerships within the community and for the good of the community.

Before we take a look at how the 4 C's relate to the realm of patient experience and patient- and family-centered care, it may be helpful to start with some definitions.

Definitions

Healthcare organizations are infamous for cooking up heaping mounds of alphabet soup: jargon and acronyms that mean something to some but not to most. My first job out of grad school was as an administrative fellow at a large tertiary hospital in Minneapolis. I'll never forget when the then-president of the foundation handed me a document that he'd found particularly helpful when he arrived. It was lovingly titled the "Abbott Northwestern Bible." In this document I found an alphabetical listing of all of the terms, acronyms, and words that meant something to those within that great institution but that could be baffling for those just entering it. That "bible" was one of the most helpful parts of my early orientation at Abbott Northwestern Hospital.

The patient satisfaction/patient experience/patient- and family-centered care space is no different. When I first got involved with work in this emerging area, it was called "patient satisfaction." Within only a few years, that term seemed outdated and was becoming more often referred to as "patient experience." According to the Centers for Medicare & Medicaid Services (CMS), from a survey perspective "patient experience surveys focus on how patients experienced or perceived key aspects of their care, not how satisfied they were with their care. Patient experience surveys focus on asking patients whether or how often they experienced critical aspects of healthcare, including communication with their doctors, understanding their medication instructions, and the coordination of their healthcare needs. They do not focus on amenities" (CMS, 2016).

In his post on the Hospital Impact blog in July 2014, Jason Wolfe, president of the Beryl Institute, wrote: "Satisfaction, the idea of how positive someone feels about an encounter, is an important metric, but experience encompasses more than just a sense of satisfaction. Satisfaction is in the moment, but experience is the lasting story. It is defined in all that is perceived, understood and remembered. And patient experience encompasses much more than creating happy patients. It is about ensuring the best in quality, safety and service outcomes."

I love the work of the Beryl Institute and have supported them and participated in their movement over the years. They define the patient experience as: "The sum of all of the interactions, shaped by the organization's culture, that influence patient perceptions across the continuum of care" (n.d.).

Fig. 1.1: Patient Experience Definition

The sum of all **interactions,** shaped by an organization's **culture,** that influence patient **perceptions** across the **continuum** of care.

- The Beryl Institute

However, I think the Beryl Institute's definition misses a key point: When I share this definition with teams and in workshops, I change it to include "patient *and family* perceptions across the continuum of care." Families are a significant factor in how patients experience their care, and therefore how they rate their care. We are increasingly hearing from patients that their family members are just as much a part of and impacted by their experiences as patients as the staff and physicians who care for them.

While the movement toward a focus on patient- and family-centered care might seem recent, the reality is that children's hospitals, perhaps the first to use the term "patient- and family-centered," have been using the term for years. The Institute for Patient- and Family-Centered Care (IFPCC) has been in existence for more than 20 years.

According to IFPCC, "Patient- and family-centered care is an approach to the planning, delivery, and evaluation of healthcare that is grounded in mutually beneficial partnerships among healthcare providers, patients, and families. It redefines the relationships in healthcare.

Patient- and family-centered practitioners recognize the vital role that families play in ensuring the health and well-being of infants, children, adolescents, and family members of all ages. They acknowledge that emotional, social, and developmental support are integral components of healthcare. They promote the health and well-being of individuals and families and restore dignity and control to them.

Patient- and family-centered care is an approach to healthcare that shapes policies, programs, facility design, and staff day-to-day interactions. It leads to better health outcomes and wiser allocation of resources, and greater patient and family satisfaction" (n.d.).

One of the earliest citations for support for patient- and family-centered care came out of the Institute of Medicine's 2001 report *Crossing the Quality Chasm: A New Health System for the 21st Century*, which, among other things, called for healthcare systems that:

- Respect patients' values, preferences, and expressed needs to be involved in their care

- Provide the information, communication, and education that people need and want

- Guarantee physical comfort, emotional support, and *the involvement of family and friends*

- Provide transformational change in healthcare

When my kids were younger, they liked to watch the PBS cartoon *Martha Speaks*. It's about a dog who eats some of the family's alphabet soup, and when she does, she can talk. To follow, let alone sort through and understand, the various definitions we've just covered feels like enough alphabet soup to keep Martha talking for a year. To understand and sift through it all, I asked a group of patient experience leaders about which terms they use in their organizations and how they would describe them. One of the best responses I received was from Brandon Parkhurst, MD, MBA, CPXP, medical director, patient experience, Marshfield Clinic (Beryl Institute Listserv):

Patient experience is defined by those receiving care (patients, families, etc.), hence it is about perception; patient-/family-centered care is defined by the intention of those providing the care (and I include both individuals and systems in the word "those"), hence it is about prioritization. In short, patient/family-centered care is a promise and patient experience is the measured outcome.

I use both terms, and I suppose that at times it might seem like I'm using them as synonyms, but I'm not. As a rule of thumb, when speaking to providers, I'll use the intention term and talk about patient-/family-centered care, as that is the primary motivation of providers ... caring for patients. When speaking to organization leaders I use the outcome term, "patient experience," as that's how we reflect upon and judge our performance. I don't see one as ever being used exclusively over the other. I see patient-/family-centeredness as a business strategy and patient experience as the measure of success.

Why should we discuss the terms within this facet of the industry, and do they even matter? Interestingly, the changes in terms have coincided with our evolving work and approach to improvement in this area. You can see on this graph how the terms "patient satisfaction" and "patient experience" have basically flip-flopped in the past 10 years, at least in terms of what is searched for on Google.

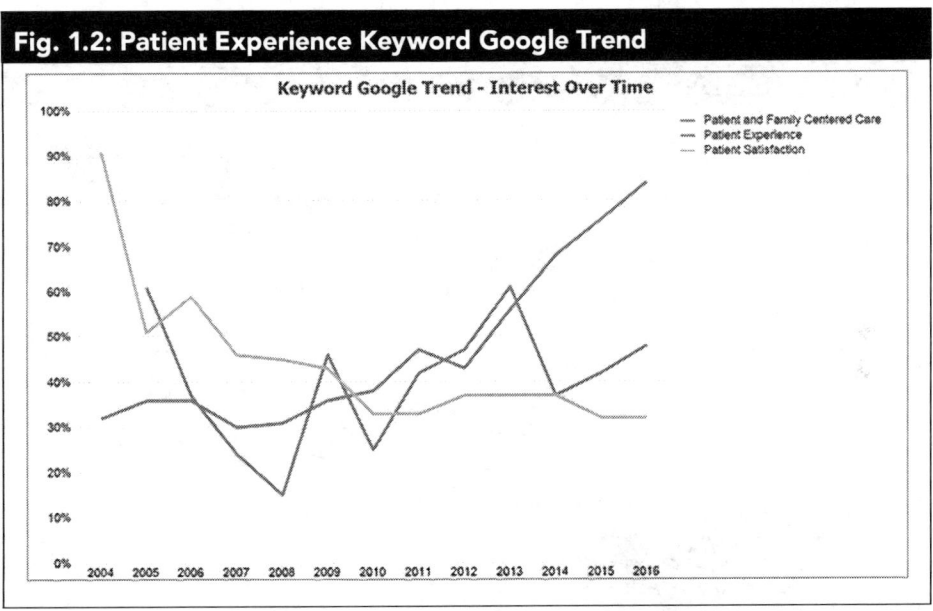

Fig. 1.2: Patient Experience Keyword Google Trend

Does it matter what you call it? I would say that it matters less what you call your work in the organization and more about how you define it. I encourage organizations to call their movement something that makes sense to the members leading it (and by members, I mean the staff and physicians as well as the executives involved with this work). I encourage organizations, whichever terms they use, to define their terms and come up with a definition that corresponds to what makes sense in their organization, similar to how you might develop a vision. For example, when working with a large Level 1 Trauma Center team at Regions Hospital in St. Paul, Minnesota, this was the definition that they created and then used throughout their training workshops with their staff:

Chapter 1

The perceptions, thoughts and feelings that patients, families and visitors have about everyone they encounter and the care they receive during their unexpected visit; from the moment they arrive throughout their care and even after they leave.

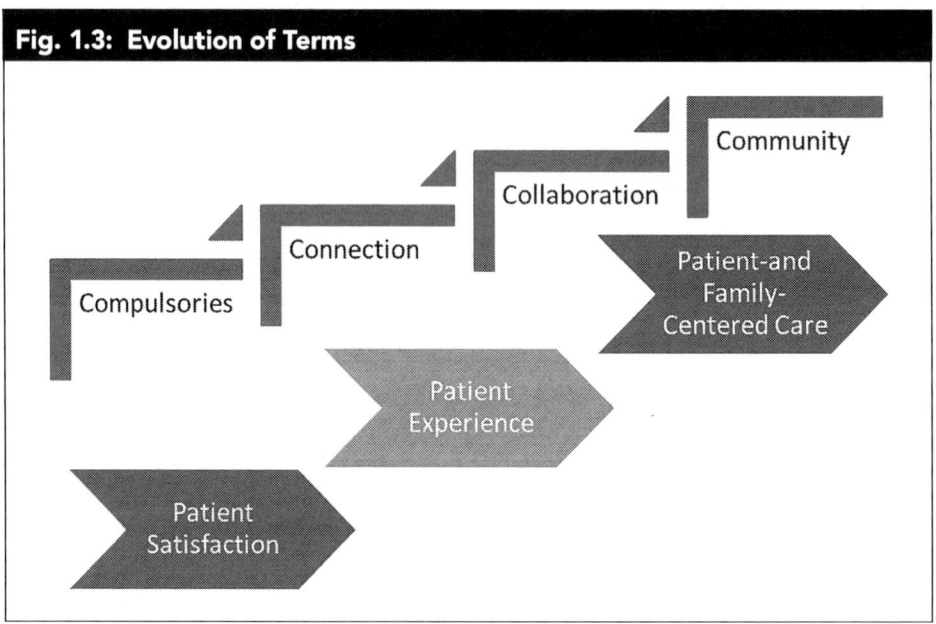

Fig. 1.3: Evolution of Terms

It was this definition, developed from a frontline interdisciplinary team, that led the group to title its workshop "The Unexpected Experience." This definition was useful to ask participants to identify which words stood out to them. The same words were heard over and over: "perceptions," "everyone," and "unexpected."

Regardless of what you call your program, it's important to have a definition of what you mean with the terms that you use and how you will know you are successful in your work. This shouldn't feel like an overwhelming or arduous task. Some of the best work I have seen is when frontline staff and physicians are paired with patients and allowed to let their creativity run free.

It's also okay to acknowledge that what your organization calls their efforts today may evolve over time. In some organizations, this seems to parallel the 4 C's model mentioned previously.

I base this on what I see in the market and the organizations that we work with; the terms seem to evolve with the approach to improvement and the entrenchment in the organization. The reality is that the bulk of organizations across the country are somewhere in their journey related to patient experience, and that's the term that seems to be most frequently used. Thus, for the balance of this book, we will use the terms "patient experience" or "patient- and family-centered care" to refer to the spectrum of these efforts, unless otherwise noted. We'll also focus on the elements of the compulsories, connection, and collaboration. Further exploration into the community and the work of patient engagement will have to be the subject of another book. For now, we have plenty to cover, so let's get started.

References

Centers for Medicare & Medicaid Services. (2016). Retrieved June 27, 2016, from *www.cms.gov/Research-Statistics-Data-and-Systems/Research/CAHPS/*

Institute for Patient- and Family-Centered Care. (n.d.). Frequently Asked Questions. Retrieved June 27, 2016, from *www.ipfcc.org/faq.html*

Institute of Medicine. (2001). Crossing the quality chasm: A new health system for the 21st century. Retrieved June 27, 2016, from *www.nap.edu/html/quality_chasm/reportbrief.pdf*

Shaller, D. (2007). Patient-centered care: What does it take? The Commonwealth Fund. Retrieved June 27, 2016, from *www.commonwealthfund.org/usr_doc/Shaller_patient-centeredcarewhatdoesittake_1067.pdf?section=4039*

The Beryl Institute. (n.d.). Defining the patient experience. Retrieved June 27, 2016, from *www.theberylinstitute.org/?page=definingpatientexp*

Wolf, J. A., Niederhauser, V., Marshburn, D., and LaVela, S. L. (2014). Defining patient experience. *Patient Experience Journal, 1*(1), Article 3. Available at *http://pxjournal.org/journal/vol1/iss1/3*. Retrieved: *http://pxjournal.org/cgi/viewcontent.cgi?article=1004&context=journal*

Parkhurst, B. (2016). Describing patient experience vs. patient- and family-centered care. PXLEADERS LISTSERV. Retrieved June 8, 2016, from *PXLEADERS@LIST.THEBERYLINSTITUTE.ORG*

Chapter 2

CAHPS = Compulsories— Necessary but Insufficient

In the last chapter, we talked about a model and approach to quality and performance improvement and started to see how it relates to the work in patient experience. Let's take a deeper look at some of the compulsories, understanding that there are many.

CMS is responsible for the development and administration of several types of patient experience surveys. These surveys are aimed at patient (and family) perceptions of their experiences across the continuum: hospitals, doctors, home health, health plans, etc. The outcomes of most of these surveys are now tied to payment in one way or another—either at a provider or a facility level.

Many of these CMS surveys are included in the family of surveys known as the CAHPS (Consumer Assessment of Health Plans and Services) surveys. These surveys are focused on aspects that are most important to patients. These aspects have been studied, and the surveys have been psychometrically tested. There are standardized questions and protocols for data collection to enable the data to be used comparatively across organizations and for benchmarking purposes (CMS, n.d.).

Chapter 2

These requirements are alive and well, and most organizations are impacted by them in at least one area of their services. Compared to when I started working in this area about eight years ago, today there's much more knowledge and understanding of the CAHPS tools, CMS requirements, and public reporting of performance. What's exciting to me is that there also seems to be recognition that CAHPS alone is not enough. Most organizations are recognizing the need to push beyond the requirements and do more than just check the box in terms of sending out surveys. That being said, it doesn't mean that everyone within those organizations easily complies with the requirements and pushes ahead to truly achieve patient- and family-centered care.

In the hospitals, clinics, and healthcare systems across the country where I get to work, I often encounter some pushback against CAHPS. Everyone fancies themselves a survey writer and many an executive knows exactly how many items should be on the survey ... 10! "Just like when I go to get my oil changed, they ask me 10 questions!" or "Maybe we should do what they do at my [insert your favorite nonhealthcare service provider], and let's give everyone a chance to win a $25 gift card to our Center for Health and Healing!" Well-meaning intentions often lead to frustrated patient experience staff trying to explain to senior leaders why these great ideas are not allowed by CMS regulation.

Being too rigid and preaching the standards and regulations of CAHPS is not a preferred position for a leader in patient experience or patient- and family-centered care. I've been there—I've told that CMO that she can't do an "enter to win a survey" scheme within the ambulatory division! And guess what? It doesn't really help your cause. So be prepared to not just tell them why they can't do what they think will help. Instead, try to harness that enthusiasm and get them to think creatively with you about what they can do.

I have friends on the CAHPS team, and I have great respect for the work that they do and the standards that have been set. I also have my own list of things that could be made better or different. I talk with them about my concerns about survey fatigue for patients and families and survey burden for organizations. And yet, I can appreciate the hard work that has gone into the public transparency and elevation of importance of the patient experience.

For many executives, they just jump to the bottom line: "So we're paying $10 to $15 per returned mail survey just to check the box on the requirements?" And then, depending on how their facility is performing, you may have this additional response:

- Bottom quartile—"We're better than that. If we just had a better response rate, then that would show up. Who fills out a paper survey that arrives via snail mail anymore anyway? This is totally biased!"

- Middle quartile—"No matter what we do, we can't seem to differentiate ourselves. The data lags on every improvement we try to make. If we just had more up-to-date data, we'd be able to do a better job of managing our process improvement around patient experience."

- Upper quartile—"See? We're the best in the community. Why do we have to keep investing in surveys to report what we already know to be true?"

Whether you're already living these conversations or you've yet to have them (and I promise you, you will!), the reality is there's so much more to this than just the scores. The challenge for those leading patient experience efforts in healthcare organizations today is that the data and the scores are only part of the story.

Tip of the Iceberg

When we talk about public transparency of the data and patient experience scores in particular, there are many people who seem to push back and hope that "this too shall pass." To them, I try to gently share a bit about the trajectory thus far.

Chapter 2

CAHPS surveying began with the health plan survey in 1997 and moved to the inpatient arena with the Hospital CAHPS (HCAHPS) in 2006. The advent of Home Health CAHPS in 2010, CAHPS for Accountable Care Organizations in 2012, In-Center Hemodialysis CAHPS (ICH CAHPS) in 2014, and Hospice CAHPS® Survey in 2015 have shown the onward march of this movement. Additionally, several states have mandated their own requirements related to the Clinician and Group (CG CAHPS) tools. For example, in my home state of Minnesota, CG CAHPS was first implemented in 2012 and is now required biannually. At the time of this writing, we are eagerly awaiting timing on the rollout of the Emergency Department Patient Experiences with Care Survey (EDPEC), and the newly released Consumer Assessment of Healthcare Providers and Systems Outpatient and Ambulatory Surgery Survey (OAS CAHPS) has just been made available for use with voluntary reporting.

Let's not forget about our friends in long-term care. CAHPS has two versions of a nursing home survey for residents—one for those who live in a nursing home and one for those who have been discharged after a short stay. Additionally, there is a family member survey for residents' families to complete.

In short, there are not many other areas across the healthcare continuum without requirements for patient experience surveys at this time. The reality is that value-based purchasing is alive and well—not just in patient experience, but in quality and outcomes as well. There is no shortage of requirements in this space. To succeed in this area, you need to be well-versed in the compulsories, keep up with them as they change, know how to navigate them, and educate others about them.

The reality is that the compulsories alone are not enough to help drive significant improvement. There are few staff, leaders, or physicians out there who are completely motivated to improve based on CAHPS requirements alone. These compulsories are necessary and have helped to elevate the focus on patient experience, but they alone will not drive improvement. Thus, I see them as necessary but insufficient to completely drive the change that organizations need to succeed in this area. In addition to mastering the compulsories, you need to also master the art of building beyond them. In the next section, we'll take a look at some of the ways to start to connect and engage the care team around meaningful improvement.

References

Agency for Healthcare Research and Quality. (2016). Clinician & group. Retrieved June 27, 2016, from *www.ahrq.gov/cahps/surveys-guidance/cg/index.html*

Agency for Healthcare Research and Quality. (2016). Development of the CAHPS health plan surveys. Retrieved June 27, 2016, from *www.ahrq.gov/cahps/surveys-guidance/hp/about/Development-CAHPS-HP-Survey.html*

Agency for Healthcare Research and Quality. (2016). Health plan survey. Retrieved June 27, 2016, from *www.ahrq.gov/cahps/surveys-guidance/hp/index.html*

Agency for Healthcare Research and Quality. (2016). Home health care. Retrieved June 27, 2016, from *www.ahrq.gov/cahps/surveys-guidance/home/index.html*

Agency for Healthcare Research and Quality. (2016). Nursing home resident surveys. Retrieved June 27, 2016, from *www.ahrq.gov/cahps/surveys-guidance/nh/resident/index.html*

Agency for Healthcare Research and Quality. (2016). Read about the health plan survey. *www.ahrq.gov/cahps/surveys-guidance/hp/about/index.html*

Centers for Medicare & Medicaid Services. (n.d.). Consumer assessment of healthcare providers & systems (CAHPS). Retrieved June 27, 2016, from *www.cms.gov/Research-Statistics-Data-and-Systems/Research/CAHPS/*

Centers for Medicare & Medicaid Services. (n.d.). CAHPS for PQRS. Retrieved June 27, 2016, from *www.cms.gov/Research-Statistics-Data-and-Systems/Research/CAHPS/pqrs.html*

Minnesota Department of Health. (2016). Data collection guide: 2016 patient experience of care measure. Retrieved June 27, 2016, from *http://mncm.org/wp-content/uploads/2015/08/2016-Patient-Exp-Data-Collection-Guide_final.pdf*

Planetree. (2012). Advancing PCC across the continuum of care. Retrieved June 27, 2016, from *www.ltlmagazine.com/sites/ltlmagazine.com/files/whitepapers/Planetree_WP_LTC-Living%20_080812.pdf*

Chapter 3
Connection to the WIIFMs—Reasons to Care

In the last chapter, we talked about the compulsories: the requirements attached to patient experience. In this section, we want to build on those and understand how they alone are not enough to motivate the care team to make significant improvements. Instead, there are a multitude of reasons to care about this work. It is essential that making the case for patient- and family-centered care extends beyond one leader, one staff member, or one department. To do this, you have to find a way to articulate the WIIFM (pronounced *wiff 'em*—what's in it for me?) for some key groups.

Depending on the audience and the role of the person you're encountering, there may be different strategies about how to make the case for patient experience. There are various methods I use to appeal to executives, physicians, and staff. I'll try to refrain from making too many stereotypes, as I find that what's compelling to one person may not be to another. However, there are some broad categories of what resonates with various groups.

There are several strategies that I use to try to approach people about why patient experience is important and why they should care about it. Broadly stated, these fall into the categories of:

Chapter 3

- What if it were me/my family?
- Employee engagement and physician satisfaction
- Financial
- Public image/transparency
- Patient activation/engagement

Rarely do I presume to start with the financial elements associated with the compulsories. To many caregivers, starting with financials is almost insulting. Most entered the healthcare profession with an innate desire to help people and make a difference in their lives. I generally try to appeal to people on a personal or even emotional level.

What If It Were Me or My Family?: Putting Yourself in the Patient's Shoes

Many caregivers have gotten disconnected from the reason that they entered the field. Many talk about how computer-based vs. people-based their work has become, and about how it is more about tasks instead of taking care of their patients. It's helpful to pull these team members away from those tasks and have them think about themselves and their loved ones. Imagining the care that they would want for themselves or the special people in their lives is one way they can reconnect with this sense of purpose and reacquaint themselves with the experiences they desire to have and to create for others.

One activity I've used to help with this is called the "Special Person Exercise." Prior to a training session, workshop, or meeting, I ask everyone attending to bring along a picture of someone who is important to them. Once they arrive, I ask them to write three words or phrases that describe that person and why they are important on a Post-It™ and put the Post-It™ on the back of the picture. Then, they bring their pictures to the front of the room and leave them there for a few moments. Usually a beautiful collage of faces and scenes emerges. And yes, there's at least one pet in every group.

Then, I ask each person in the room to come up and grab a photo that is not their own. Using these photos as part of our introduction, we go around the room having each person stand up, introduce him- or herself, and show the photo that he or she selected. He or she reads the three words that are written on the back of the photo, and then I ask him or her to say why he or she chose that photo off of the wall. What drew the person to select it? By this, each person makes connections. Sometimes it's a "Well, this little guy had a Twins hat on, and I love baseball." Or "She had lovely eyes" or "This puppy reminded me of the dog I had growing up."

Once done, he or she asks the person who brought that photo to stand up, and then that person shares the photo that he or she selected off the wall, and so on. This is a powerful exercise—one that often leads to laughter, and sometimes even a few tears.

Why do I do that? Why would I "waste" valuable caregivers' time in a meeting or workshop to do this? I see this as a great centering activity for a group. It helps to remind us that each and every one of us has special people in our lives. When we can realize that all of the patients who come to our clinic, our hospital, our lab, our nursing home, our urgent care, or our ED are special to someone, it can change how we approach them. When we remember that everyone is special to someone and think about how we'd want our special people to be treated, it can make a big difference.

Sometimes, depending on the care setting and the situation, it's quite possible that the person we're caring for no longer has someone who would consider him or her their "special person." I was reminded of this when working in a Level 1 Trauma Center in a large urban hospital. The staff there talked about the people that they care for—many of them homeless and without a support network. One nurse said to me, "I try to remember that they may not have a special person, but for that moment, I can be that for them. I can care for them like I would my own brother, mother, friend."

This is profound and something that requires much empathy and mindfulness. It's tough to keep this mindset each and every day depending on what all we may have going on in our own lives—work and personal.

Employee Engagement and Physician Satisfaction

I also try to connect staff and providers with the idea of their own engagement in the care they provide. Yes, some are motivated by thinking about the care they would want for themselves and their loved ones. As one social worker said, "I try to remember 'There but for the grace of God go I.' It could be my family member or me."

For others, though, there's another aspect that resonates, and it's the pride they feel about the work they do. Many feel like they spend more time at work than they do at home with the special people in their lives. They have worked hard and spent many years investing in their education and training. When they go home after their shift, how do they feel? Did they provide the best care possible that day?

There are times that I encounter some pushback from staff and providers in the form of "What about us?" Often there's been too much focus on patient experience and "the numbers," to the exclusion of the team, such that they become jaded and the meaning behind the patient experience becomes lost on the staff and providers. One nurse said to me: "Don't talk to me about patient experience until we've talked about the staff experience."

And you know what? She was right. Organizations are making a mistake when they push staff to focus more on the patients and families without doing enough to acknowledge staff and provider satisfaction and experience. In addition to patient experience data, it's imperative to pay attention to some other key sources of data in the organization, especially the employee engagement and physician satisfaction scores.

When thinking about the WIIFM around patient experience related to staff and providers, it's important that organizations pay attention to the tools and support that their teams need to provide the best care possible to the patients and families entrusting them with their care.

The Financial Component

For some, the financial component of patient experience is compelling. Although I don't usually start with this argument, it is something that is important to certain groups. I'm often surprised which ones. For example, when working with an interdisciplinary team of staff and physicians at a large Level 1 Trauma Center, I shared a bit about how patient experience factors into value-based purchasing. My assumption was that they wouldn't want to include this in a workshop for their department and that we would emphasize other aspects of why focusing on patient experience was important instead. However, they totally surprised me. They saw this video on YouTube that my team, DTA Associates, had created and they insisted that we share it in their upcoming workshop for all staff.

Chapter 3

Fig. 3.1: Value-Based Purchasing

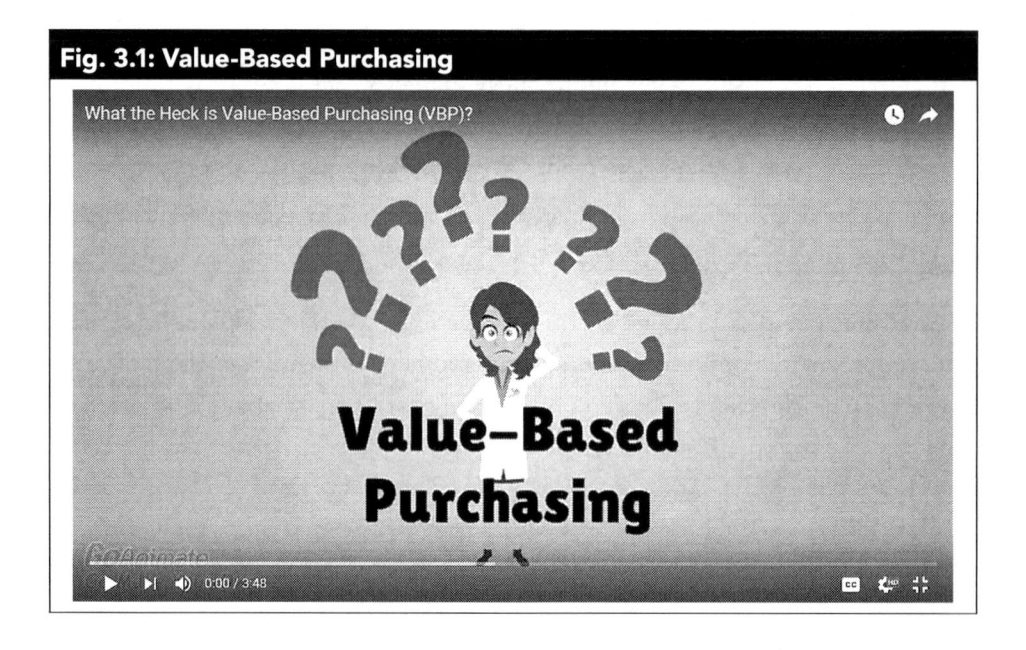

One nurse said, "I think it's important; our team needs to understand that this impacts how we get paid, and that translates into the resources available within the department. Plus, it's available to the public. I want them to know how we're going to be perceived in the community." So we shared this component, and it was helpful to that department. Most people had no idea that this was impacting the hospital, let alone their department.

Like I said, I'm often surprised about with whom this aspect does and does not connect—the ED staff wanted to include it, but some hospital presidents hardly bat an eye at the financial elements. One president of a prominent urban tertiary hospital said to me, "Four hundred thousand dollars isn't really a blip on my radar." In large organizations, the financial element of CMS' value-based purchasing is not always enough to really get their attention.

If we look only at CMS and their component of this financial equation, that may be true. However, in our work in quality and patient experience, as well as our work with the payer community, we've always advocated for aligned incentives. In that same organization where the hospital president bluntly shared that $400,000 wasn't a big number to him, there were also several payer contracts with similar incentives that amounted to upward of $1,000,000 for achieving certain quality and patient experience goals.

Whether initiated by the organization or the payer, we see more alignment in these key quality and outcome measures. The payer community is watching what CMS is doing and is following suit with their contracts as well.

For many staff and physicians who we work with, the financial element is not the most compelling part of patient experience. Depending on their affiliation and relationship (employed or not) with a hospital or healthcare organization, the physicians may see this as something for the hospitals to worry about, but not for themselves to worry about. Yet for others, they see the bigger picture and how this impacts the scarce resources across the healthcare continuum, and they want to maximize that which is at their and their organization's disposal.

Our team was working with an interdisciplinary group of physicians, nurses, techs, health unit coordinators, social workers, police officers, and other staff in a large urban area. We were talking about patient experience and what was important about it, and what resonated most with the teams in their areas. I was blown away by a nurse who spoke up and said, "Well, isn't this tied to our payments and how much we make as a hospital? I think people need to know about that. We don't need to make them experts, but they should know something about the reality of what our hospital is facing."

Public Image and Transparency

Slightly related and yet somewhat tangential to the financial conversation is the aspect of public transparency and the prestige or image of the healthcare organization. This is another aspect I find many CEOs and other leaders respond to, as well as many physicians and frontline staff. Appealing to the

Chapter 3

competitive nature of many of these people is another way to get buy-in for the work and focus in patient experience.

Let's face it: Healthcare is a competitive industry. In recent years there has been (and will continue to be) increasing consolidation in the marketplace. With this, there is heightened competition between a smaller number of providers. There are some exceptions, but most people want to work for "the best."

When the CAHPS, Net Promoter, or any other scores are published online, many patients and consumers pay attention to them, but many staff within those organizations do as well. Again, this is not an aspect that I dwell on too much, but I like to leverage that sense of healthy competition.

In a workshop in California with frontline staff, we pulled up the Hospital Compare website and showed that particular hospital's scores. We then proceeded to show them scores from their competitors in the nearby city, and then asked the participants to describe their performance relative to the others. It was a fun and engaging way to get the participants connected to caring about this in a new way. They had their opinions about the other local facilities (many of them were worse than their employer, of course). Yet when they saw the scores as reported by actual patients, they were astounded and a little offended. Again, they felt like they'd chosen to work at the best place and they believed that they provided the best care, and yet they didn't really see that reflected in the scores; this helped them articulate that they wanted to see something different. My favorite description was one nursing assistant who raised his hand and said that relative to the local competitors, he'd describe this hospital's performance as "middleish."

Physicians are particularly competitive, and this is also a fun way to engage them in the public image of what's out there for their patients to see. These types of discussions are helpful and engaging to appeal to that sense of employee engagement where we want to be giving our time and want to work at the best place possible.

When I was working with a frontline nursing team in a cardiac unit of a tertiary urban hospital, we were talking about the data, the scores, and public transparency. This was new to many of the nurses on the team. Some were inclined to not dwell on it until one nurse spoke up. She shared the story of a conversation she'd recently had with her father who was in his late 60s and in need of knee surgery. She was telling him about her project and what she'd been learning about public transparency, etc. He said, "Oh yeah, I've heard of that. I went on to Hospital Compare to look at the facilities in my area before I decided where to go for my knee surgery." This woman was shocked that her father knew about this before she did, and he had even used it to help make his decisions!

National tools and survey scores are just one way to look at the community's perceptions about the organization. It is also really important to think about the other measures of the perception of the organization, many of which can be determined via social media. I often refer to these as the informal measures of patient experience. Whether it is Yelp, Facebook, Twitter, Glassdoor, Reputation.com, or Angie's List, there are many other places and sources of data for potential patients to consider when looking for information about the organizations in their area. It's increasingly important that those leading patient experience efforts within the organization are focused on informal measures of patient experience. Often those coordinating and responding to the organization's social media presence are housed in the marketing and communications area, so connections with those departments are critical to the patient experience leader's success.

Chapter 3

Connection Between Patient Experience and Patient Engagement

More than just semantics, there is a difference between patient experience and patient engagement—and a connection, too.

I see patient engagement as the top rung of the patient experience ladder. For many patients, it is only when they feel like they have been treated with courtesy and respect, and have been listened to carefully, that they are able to truly "hear" their providers. When they do hear, it's imperative that those providers are explaining things in a way that they can understand. It's only when these key communication elements of patient experience are consistently achieved that we are able to actually engage patients in their own care.

This is the aspect where physicians get "hooked." I can't tell you how many physicians who I work with totally get that care within the walls of a traditional healthcare system comprises only 10% of a person's determinants of health (see Figure 3.2).

They fully acknowledge that we are one small piece of the puzzle for patients. The reality is that so much more (30%–40%) is within their patients' control and doesn't intersect directly with a hospital at all. Things like medication adherence and lifestyle choices have just as big of an impact on outcomes, if not more, as care provided in the hospital or clinic. When we talk about the fact that a good patient experience leads to higher patient engagement, we are then able to get the attention of many of the physicians (Community Health).

Fig. 3.2: Determinants of Health

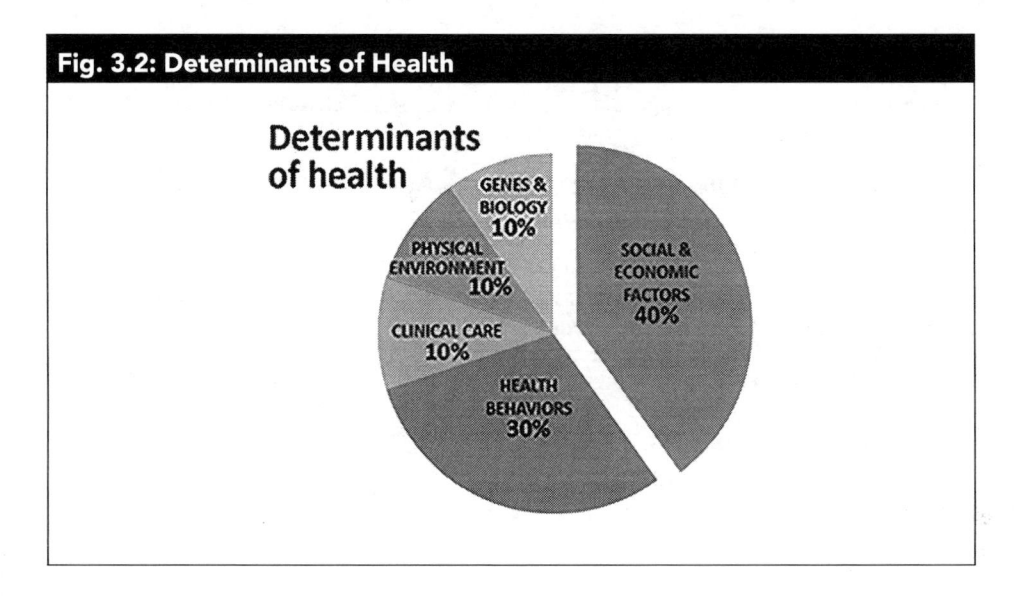

Determinants of health
- GENES & BIOLOGY 10%
- PHYSICAL ENVIRONMENT 10%
- SOCIAL & ECONOMIC FACTORS 40%
- CLINICAL CARE 10%
- HEALTH BEHAVIORS 30%

Depending on the culture and composition of your organization, you may have to deploy many or even all of these strategies to connect and engage staff, physicians, and leaders. Remember that there are compelling ways to talk about the various WIIFMs (McGinnis, Williams-Russo, & Krickman, 2002; Tarlov, 1999):

- What if it were me/my family?

- Employee engagement and physician satisfaction

- Financial

- Public image/transparency

- Patient activation/engagement

It's important to feel well-prepared for the various perspectives you may encounter across the organization. Success is found by those who have a variety of approaches to meet these varied stakeholders and opinions. One of the best starting points for pursuing connection and engagement with the care team is starting with the patients. We'll explore that next.

References

Center for Health and Learning. (n.d.). Community health. Retrieved June 27, 2016, from *https://healthandlearning.org/community-health/*

DTA Associates, Inc. (2014). *What the Heck Is Value-Based Purchasing?* [online video] Retrieved June 27, 2016, from *www.youtube.com/watch?v=dF8SGblP7-c*

McGinnis, J. M., Williams-Russo, P., and Knickman, J. R. (2002). The case for more active policy attention to health promotion. *Health Affairs*, 21(2), 78–93. Retrieved June 27, 2016, from *http://content.healthaffairs.org/content/21/2/78.long*

Tarlov, A. R. (1999). Public policy frameworks for improving population health. Ann N Y Acad Sci 1999; 896: 281-93. Retrieved June 27, 2016, from *www.ncbi.nlm.nih.gov/pubmed/10681904*.

Section 2

Foundation/Connection and Collaboration—Patients and People

Chapter 4
Patients Are the Reason We Exist

Once we understand the compulsories and can establish the WIIFMs (What's in it for Me?) to care about patient experience, then we can actually start to engage the various stakeholders in the work of improving the experiences of patients and families. One of the best ways to do this is to project the voices of those very patients and families.

When I was helping to design and build an ambulatory center in 2002, we thought we were very advanced. We wanted to make sure that it really embodied a "healing environment." The center was beautiful, with wetland paths surrounding it, a water feature in the main lobby, carefully chosen color palettes, soothing sounds piped in through the ceiling, elimination of overhead paging, windows to view the wetlands, beautiful artwork—all with the intent of creating a healing environment.

We even painstakingly walked through functional flow assessments for each and every clinic and outpatient space. With the assistance of an industrial engineer, we created what we thought would be the ideal flow and process for both the staff and the patients. While we pulled in key staff members with expertise in lab, radiology, cardiology, internal medicine, surgery centers, etc., we never once pulled in a patient to help with the design. Each of us thought that by putting our own patient hat on and thinking of our friends and family members and what they would want, we'd have it nailed. We did do a focus group of patients (using a two-way mirror) and asked them about what they wanted in an orthopedic surgery center, but that's as far as we went. It never occurred to us to solicit one of those patients from the marketing focus group to actually join us in the design phase.

However, most performance improvement methodologies put the patient or the customer in the driver's seat of the intended change. For example, Lean/Six Sigma methodology starts with the voice of the customer, understands customer requirements, and then maps the current state process from a customer's vantage point. Then, future state processes are designed that eliminate non-value-added steps (from the customer perspective) and better match customers' requirements. I remember clearly when I was first being trained in Lean/Six Sigma, we were told to start with the voice of the customer, but instead we sort of laughed and said, "Yeah, how are we going to get the patients to talk to us about this?" At that time (it was 2005, so not that long ago), we all kind of laughed about how that would never happen. We did our very best to just guess what we thought they wanted and what we would want if we were patients, and built from there.

I look back on these experiences now and think how shortsighted we were. We didn't know exactly how to pull the patients in, but we knew we should have. I regret that we didn't push harder to figure out how to incorporate them into those projects and sessions. These two experiences have greatly shaped and challenged me in the work I engage in today. Sometimes our failures are our greatest teachers. It's because of this that I'm so passionate about incorporating the voices of our patients and family members into all of the work that we do. There are various ways to do so; let's look at a few of the most common ways.

Patient and Family Advisory Councils

One of the first things we created when developing the patient experience program at Allina Health was the Patient and Family Advisory Council (PFAC). This was in early 2009, and we looked to the models from Dana-Farber Cancer Institute and a few others to help guide us. Fortunately, today there are many resources available to help you get started with these groups.

There are many reasons to create a PFAC in your organization, but there are also some really important aspects to consider when you do so. Whenever an organization is looking to start a PFAC, I really push the leaders to articulate what they hope to accomplish by having one. You'd be surprised by the number of organizations, service lines within an organization, or departments within an organization that can't really answer what they are hoping to accomplish. They know they need a PFAC or they think they might need one and they haven't gotten further than that. For many, it almost seemed like it was cool or the trend to have one. Often once they developed it, however, the issue became, "Okay, now what?"

Most performance improvement methodologies insist on always having a charter. And while I know that in theory, I'm not always a huge stickler for them. However, the PFAC is one definite exception. I find it absolutely imperative for the organization to develop its own position paper/charter as to why it wants to create a PFAC and how it will use the council. In this, it's important to develop the structure for how the group will be organized and supported, where the group members' feedback will flow within the organization, which committees will oversee their work, and how their voices will be incorporated into actual change within the organization.

I consult with organizations to develop the criteria by which an agenda item goes to the PFAC. What are we asking the patients and families, and will we be able to make changes based on the feedback that they give us? We learned this the hard way early on with one of the first PFACs that we started at

Allina Health. It was within the breast program of the oncology service line. There was an amazing group of committed women who came together on a bimonthly basis to advise the breast program committee on key aspects of their clinical and program agenda. After the first year, one of the team members supporting this PFAC tallied up over 52 items that the patients had given as suggestions.

In this instance, the structure and flow of the PFAC was well articulated. Two members of the PFAC attended each breast program committee meeting; they were always first on the agenda, and they had the close attention of the physicians and other care team members leading breast cancer improvement work across the system. What wasn't well developed was a vetting process and a staged improvement trajectory to make the most of those patients' feedback and time. In the gleeful excitement of having the first PFAC and this passionate group of patients who wanted to give their voices to help make a difference, the agendas had become "What do you think about this?" "What do you think we should do about that?" and so on.

At the end of that first year, the organization realized, as did the patients, that there was no way that action could be taken on all of the 52 aspects that had been suggested. This PFAC decided to meet less often (quarterly), and the clinical service line became more strategic in how it approached the PFAC to make the best use of everyone's precious time.

Despite all of this, however, one of my favorite stories was of a meaningful change that this PFAC had on the clinical plan for improvement for the breast program committee. The committee was looking at the various cycle times between detection and treatment outcomes. It was identifying an area of focus for the next year as part of its annual goal-setting process. The committee took this to the PFAC and asked the members to weigh in on which distinct aspects of the journey were most important to them. The patients identified that minimizing the amount of time between the screening mammogram and the diagnostic mammogram was the most important to them.

The providers and care team members were floored, and pointed out that the amount of time between the screening and diagnostic mammograms made absolutely no difference from a clinical perspective and in the treatment or in outcomes. But when they heard from the patients about the sleepless nights caused by waiting and wondering if they really did have breast cancer, the committee undertook an initiative to reduce the amount of time patients had to wait for the more definitive answer of a diagnostic mammogram. Everyone was delighted when they were able to decrease that time from screening to diagnostic mammography and get it as close to the same day as possible across the system!

I love stories like this, of key successes that make a difference in the lives of patients and their families, and are so out of the realm of where healthcare organizations would be drawn to focus due to the simple fact that they are not patients. This is emblematic of some of the greatest accomplishments that organizations can make when they truly engage their patient and family advisors in the improvement process.

Getting started

There are many different models of what people consider to be a PFAC, everything from a focus group to a partnership with clinicians and staff. It's important to ensure that whatever you take to the PFAC is truly actionable and not just something you're asking the PFAC to "rubber stamp." The work that you bring to them also needs to be paced. As in the breast program committee example above, you need to be thoughtful about how much you take to them and what is truly able to be realized in a given time frame.

It's also really important that the PFAC and its feedback not exist in a vacuum. Whatever you call the group in your organization and whatever their main purpose (e.g., patient experience, safety), there needs to be a clear path of where their feedback is shared. Too often, I encounter organizations where the PFAC meets and gives insight into some key aspects of care, and the

Chapter 4

only people who see this are the patient experience people or the team that requested the information and feedback from the PFAC. I advocate strongly that the PFAC have a reporting path to another oversight group within the organization, and not just that they report there, but that one or two representatives of the PFAC actually sit on that oversight group.

In the breast program PFAC referenced earlier, two members of that group sat on the breast program committee. As the first item on the agenda, they shared a few summary slides about what they talked about at the last meeting. Obviously, picking the right PFAC members who can sit in on these meetings and represent the group is important. In other settings where we've had a PFAC with a focus on patient experience, we've had one to two members sit on the systemwide Patient Experience Steering team with the physicians, nursing leaders, and executives leading the patient experience improvement work.

Here are a few examples from other organizations' PFAC structures:

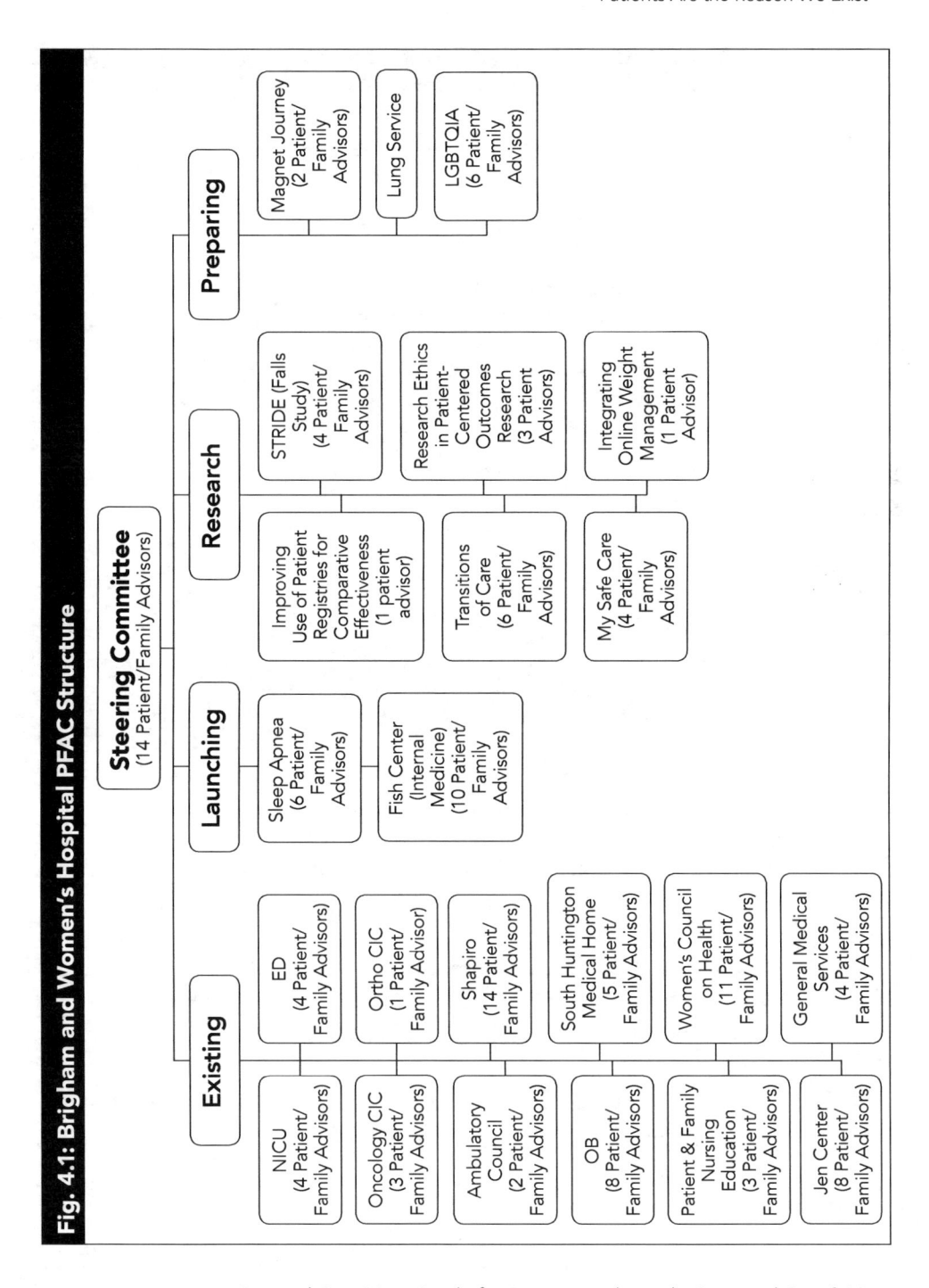

Patients Are the Reason We Exist

Fig. 4.1: Brigham and Women's Hospital PFAC Structure

Steering Committee
(14 Patient/Family Advisors)

Existing
- ED (4 Patient/Family Advisors)
  - NICU (4 Patient/Family Advisors)
- Ortho CIC (1 Patient/Family Advisor)
  - Oncology CIC (3 Patient/Family Advisors)
- Shapiro (14 Patient/Family Advisors)
  - Ambulatory Council (2 Patient/Family Advisors)
- South Huntington Medical Home (5 Patient/Family Advisors)
  - OB (8 Patient/Family Advisors)
- Women's Council on Health (11 Patient/Family Advisors)
  - Patient & Family Nursing Education (3 Patient/Family Advisors)
- General Medical Services (4 Patient/Family Advisors)
  - Jen Center (8 Patient/Family Advisors)

Launching
- Sleep Apnea (6 Patient/Family Advisors)
- Fish Center (Internal Medicine) (10 Patient/Family Advisors)

Research
- STRIDE (Falls Study) (4 Patient/Family Advisors)
  - Improving Use of Patient Registries for Comparative Effectiveness (1 patient advisor)
- Research Ethics in Patient-Centered Outcomes Research (3 Patient Advisors)
  - Transitions of Care (6 Patient/Family Advisors)
- Integrating Online Weight Management (1 Patient Advisor)
  - My Safe Care (4 Patient/Family Advisors)

Preparing
- Magnet Journey (2 Patient/Family Advisors)
- Lung Service
- LGBTQIA (6 Patient/Family Advisors)

© 2016 HCPro   Beyond CAHPS: A Guide for Patient- and Family-Centered Care | **39**

Chapter 4

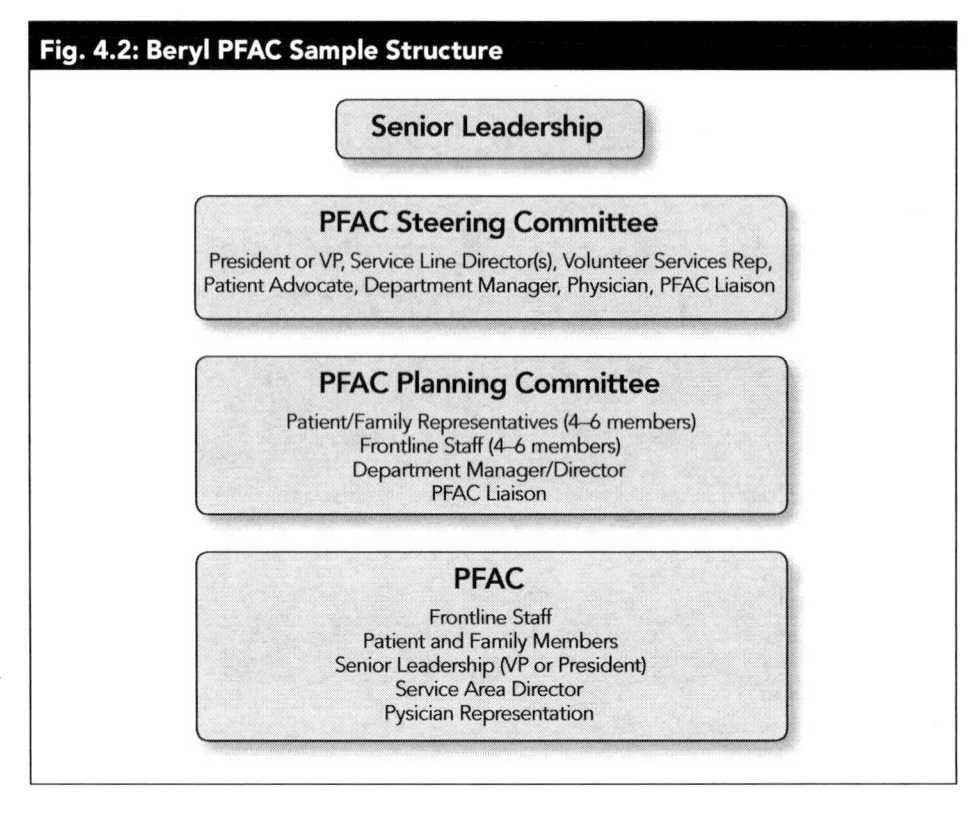

Fig. 4.2: Beryl PFAC Sample Structure

Senior Leadership

PFAC Steering Committee
President or VP, Service Line Director(s), Volunteer Services Rep, Patient Advocate, Department Manager, Physician, PFAC Liaison

PFAC Planning Committee
Patient/Family Representatives (4–6 members)
Frontline Staff (4–6 members)
Department Manager/Director
PFAC Liaison

PFAC
Frontline Staff
Patient and Family Members
Senior Leadership (VP or President)
Service Area Director
Pysician Representation

Regardless of your specific structure, having these members sit on the broader oversight group for their area of focus serves two purposes:

1. It allows the patients and family members to know that their feedback has been delivered to and heard by the leaders of their focus area.

2. It keeps those leaders grounded in the voices of their patients and families. Starting a meeting with those patient voices and stories right away helps to center and ground the purpose.

I liken this to how many religiously affiliated organizations will start a meeting with prayer or invocation. Starting with the patient and family voices helps to put everything else in the meeting into the proper perspective.

Even beyond the PFAC liaison members sharing with their oversight committee, I also advocate for a clear communication plan for dissemination of their feedback. I've helped organizations develop their communications cascade of where all those patient voices can be shared. One way to help facilitate this is by having an observer/recorder at the PFAC help distill the information into four to six PowerPoint slides as a talking point summary. This can then be used with the oversight committee but then can also be shared with other applicable groups.

Virtual PFACs and e-advisors

An increasing number of hospitals and health systems are looking at some virtual models for how to incorporate patient and family feedback. The first time I heard about this was with an organization that was going through its patient portal implementation. This particular organization included an opt-in mechanism for patients so that as they signed up for the portal, they could indicate if they were willing to be contacted as part of a virtual patient feedback group. They could specify which issues or areas they'd like to be included in (e.g., women's health, cancer care), and through this the organization was able to enlist thousands of patients and families to provide feedback on a wide array of issues. The names were pulled into a database that the organization was then able to query based on what type of feedback it needed. It could stratify by age or other demographic information, geography, and area of expertise. For instance, if it wanted to open up a new dialysis center in a certain part of the city, it could easily identify patients and families in that area with a connection to that service. It could then ask these specific people for their input on the development or other key aspects of consideration.

Organizations like University of Michigan Health System and Nemours Children's Health System have had tremendous success with the use of e-advisors and virtual PFACs. Not only are these and other hospitals using Facebook, Twitter, and other forms of social media to recruit patients and families as advisors, but they are also finding that these vehicles can provide more opportunity for feedback than the traditional patient and family council structures (Landro, 2013).

The benefits of virtual PFACs and e-advisors are numerable, including:

- Ability for patients and families to provide feedback anytime, anywhere, when it is most convenient for them
- Removal of time and geographic barriers
- Lower cost than in-person meetings and less resource-intensive in terms of staff and logistics
- Greater diversity in advisor participation
- More frequent and timely feedback

Patient comments

PFACs are some of the more robust and resource-intensive ways to gather patient feedback and input. At the other end of the spectrum, don't forget about something you already have: patient comments from patient surveys. This is one way to make the compulsories work for you. For all of the arguments that patient experience quantitative data may receive, the biggest underutilized resource is in the qualitative comments that are provided via patient comments on surveys. Again, the words of the patients and families are often the most compelling to caregivers. Finding ways to distribute these to them in a regular and personalized fashion is of utmost importance.

When I was leading work focused on physician communication improvement in patient experience, we created the Hospital Outstanding Patient Experience (HOPE) award. Every time that physicians were named positively in a patient comment, they received a certificate signed by the president of the hospital and the vice president of medical affairs (VPMA). They also received a letter signed by the VPMA listing the exact patient comment. A copy of this letter was put in the physician's file in the Medical Affairs office. At the end of the year, all of the HOPE award recipients were invited to a dinner.

In another variation of this, one vice president of medical quality sent a handwritten thank-you note to each physician who was named positively in a patient comment. Depending on the size of your organization, this may seem like a daunting task. However, I can tell you that it is not only possible but very powerful, to incorporate this even in the largest of organizations.

This doesn't just apply to physicians: One ED we worked with was able to get its discharge phone call data and patient comments stratified by the nurse and physician who cared for those patients. The ED would send these comments to them via email each week. In addition, these comments were collated annually and incorporated into performance evaluations.

Another good idea is starting each team huddle with a positive patient comment. This is a great way to send the team out into their shift. Nursing teams that I've worked with have gotten creative and made word clouds of their patient comments to post in the break room or the bathroom (the place you want to post things that you really want to get read!).

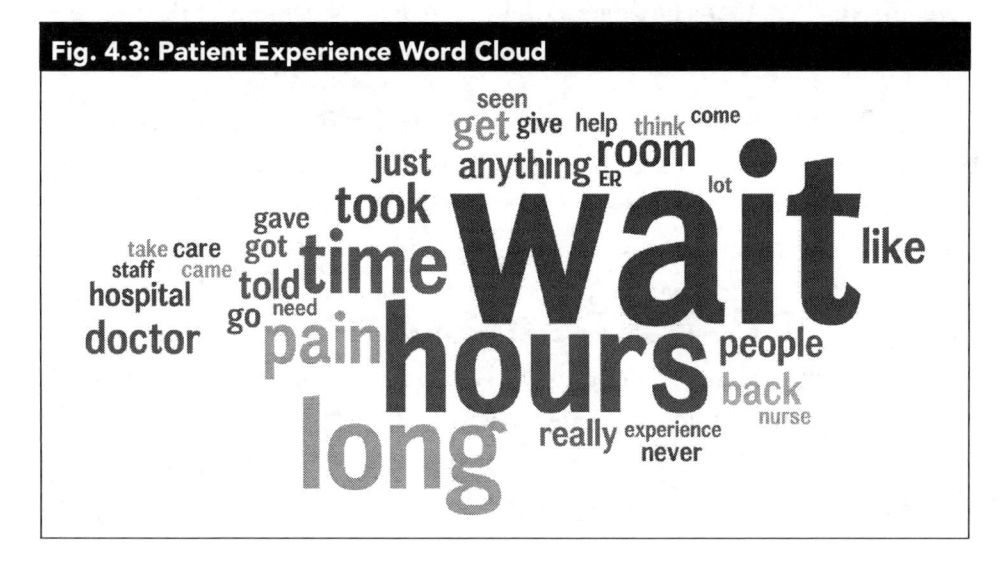

Fig. 4.3: Patient Experience Word Cloud

Many of the survey vendors will categorize the patient comments when they are transcribed into the reporting system. This makes it easy to pull the comments based on themes like pain management, communication, medications, responsiveness, coordination, etc.

I once had a patient experience department of six (yes, six) performance improvement managers. We took this practice to heart and made sure that we started our team meetings with patient comments and stories, too. The people working in this area need that same reinforcement and grounding as the frontline staff. Furthermore, for us, it was great to help emulate and really practice what we preached across the organization.

We'll spend more time on data in subsequent chapters, but I strongly encourage organizations to not show their quantitative scores in reports without making sure to include some qualitative comments alongside them. For example, with one organization we had a focus on environmental cleanliness. We created a flash report to show the numeric values and trends within that organization. On that same report, there were patient comments that related to both strengths and opportunities of cleanliness as examples.

One of my favorite things about patient comments is the ability to use them to tell a story. We've developed several exercises in which we take a real patient comment from the organization or unit we are working with and pair it with a plausible patient story. The way we use the exercise is to show a photo on the screen and have someone read the patient comment. Then we have someone read the patient story. The stories are basically some creative writing based on what could be a possible backstory to that comment. This is a powerful way to help bring patient comments to life for staff.

Consider these examples:

Example #1

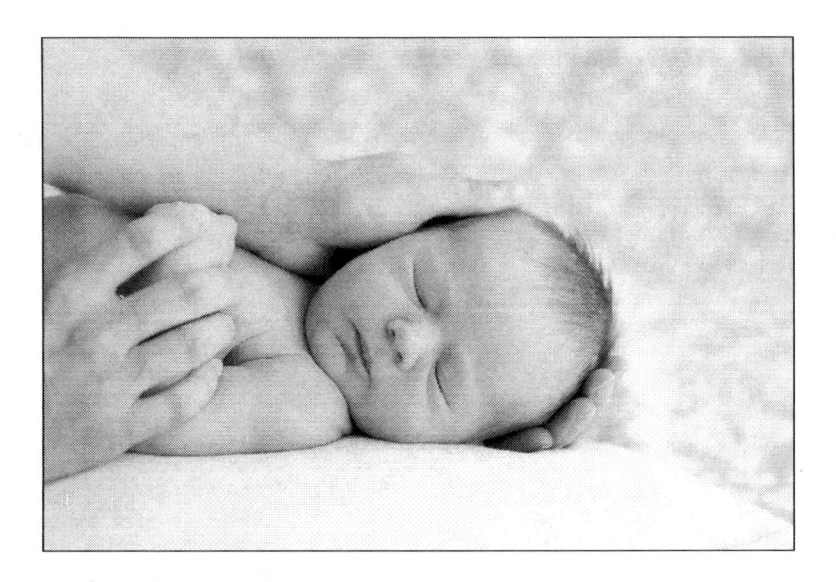

Patient comment: *All the physicians were great. The rapid response team could tell I was worried, and they helped calm me down and explain what was going on. Dr. Smith is a wonderful physician. Staff was very professional and caring. They were genuinely concerned for the well-being of our child. They answered our questions, followed up on our calls, and made a difficult situation a little bit better.*

It was so nice to have the free accommodations, the last two days of his stay, for breastfeeding purposes. It was very appreciated!! They also provided very helpful recommendations for care after taking him home. The lactation department also provided a lot of help!! These people were part of saving our son's life and protecting his brain development. Thank you will never be enough!

Patient story: *I'll never forget the day my water broke ... six weeks earlier than anticipated, while standing at my desk talking to my boss who had just popped her head in to say "Good night!" My mind could not fathom what was happening—so*

Chapter 4

soon, and I was so unprepared. This was not the way I'd anticipated this happening, not without Matt here with me. Shouldn't I be at home? Forget the meeting tomorrow; forget that nothing was ready for me to be out on leave, nothing was ready with the nursery. What now?

My husband Matt and I found each other later in life, so I was 39 when I got pregnant. When everything was happening so fast, so early, so sudden, I was petrified … would we lose this opportunity, which may be one of our last shots at having a family?

Example #2

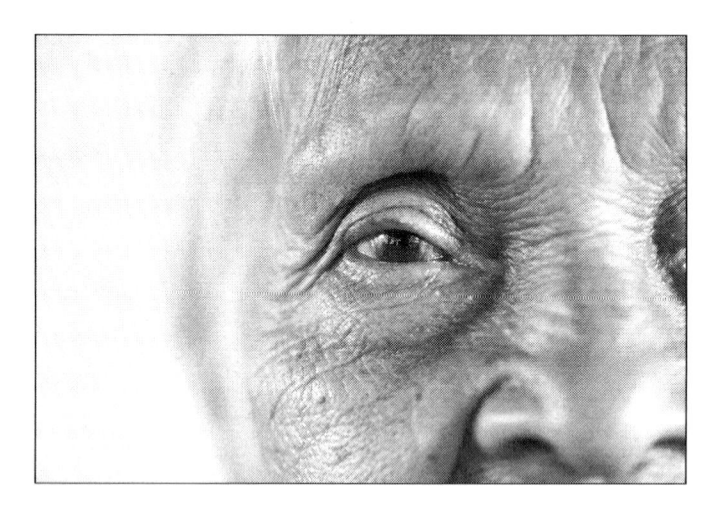

Patient comment: *I had no help when after diagnosed with a kidney stone that I was supposed to release on my own. I had no help getting to the bathroom. I had to unplug my own needle and meds to go to the bathroom by myself. It was very hard!*

Patient story: *I guess you'd say I'm what they call "fiercely independent," or at least that's what I would have said before this week. Phew, never experienced pain like this except when I had my daughter, Michelle, more than 40 years ago. And unlike that experience, where my husband, Joe, was right there with me, here I* was, without him, all alone. Joe's been gone for two years now, taken from me way too soon and too young.

And my Michelle, I'm so proud of her, she's got that big job out in California, wants me to move out there to be closer to her. But, "I'm just fine right here," that's what I told her. After this experience, I'm not so sure.

Example #3

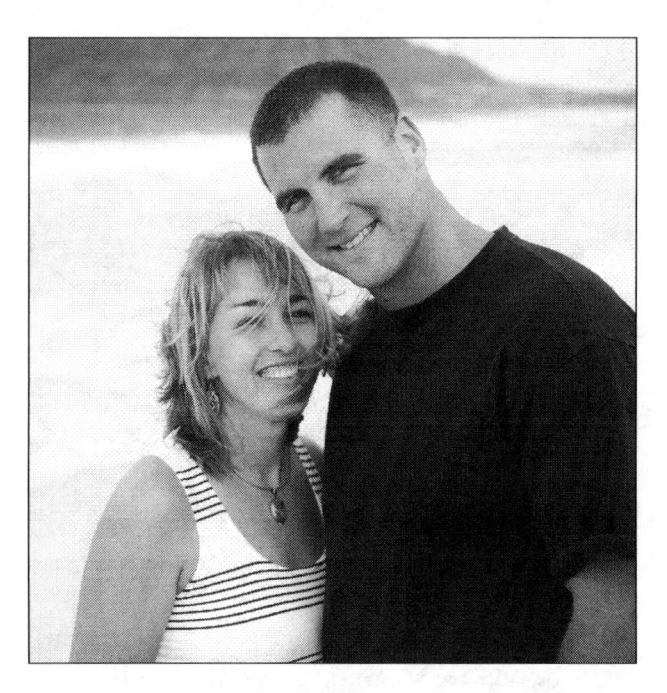

Patient comment: *Keeping track of all of my outpatient appointments and therapy has been difficult. We are so thankful for the staff at our primary care clinic in Woodbury for helping to keep us organized and moving through the process. Without their help and coordination, we would not have made it through this.*

Patient story: *It was our two-year wedding anniversary, so to celebrate, Kala and I decided to go skiing and reminisce how and where we first met. I've been skiing since I was little, and I'm fairly good. But for whatever the reason, that day, I took a jump a little off kilter, and bam! I was down and knocked out.*

Chapter 4

I can't imagine how Kala kept it together, as she was skiing behind me and saw the whole thing happen, with me landing facedown in the snow.

The next thing I knew I was in and out in the ambulance, I guess, with Kala's face swimming in and out of focus. Then, I woke up in the hospital. My lovely bride, this was not at all how we were to spend our weekend.

Since then, nothing has been normal. Kala has barely been back to work with taking me to all of my appointments and helping with the kids. They say if I'm lucky I'll get to return to teaching but probably not till next semester.

Example #4

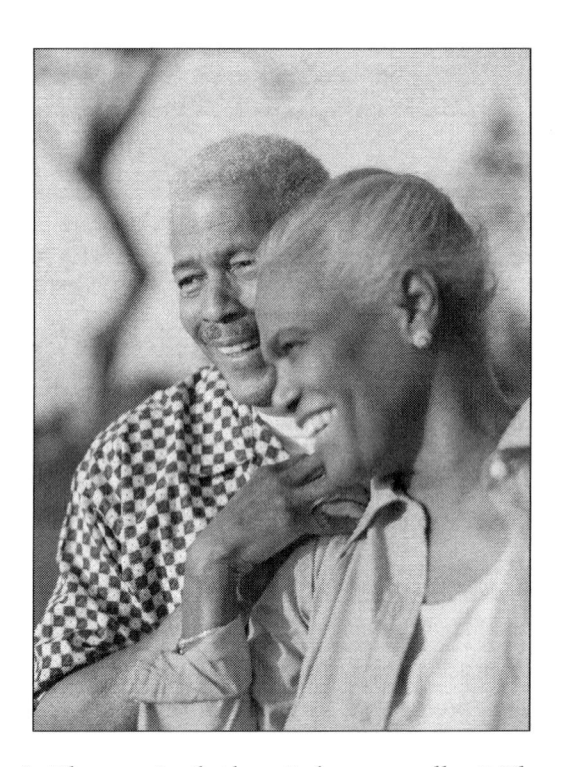

Patient comment: *The care in the hospital was excellent! The care on the main floor rehab unit was just okay. We hardly ever saw the nurse, and I had soiled my pants one morning and no one noticed or bothered to clean me up. My wife had to clean me when she arrived.*

Patient story: *My name is John, and my beautiful wife, Kathy, of 45 years and I have been enjoying our golden years together. We love to spend time up at our lake home in northern Minnesota, and we never miss the opportunity to watch the sunset together over the lake. Together we still love to attend our weekly card games, attend our weekly church services, volunteer at the local food shelf, as well as many other activities together. Recently, we became proud grandparents of our sixth grandchild.*

Unfortunately, my health has taken a turn for the worse with my hip surgery and subsequent infections; yes, plural. I try not to let it slow me down. I really worry about how my health will affect my ability to take care of Kathy. She is a proud cancer survivor of 10 years but needs my help with many of her medications and other daily activities. I worry about caring for her when I'm stuck here in this rehab unit, trying to get well.

I encourage you to consider finding ways to get creative and help bring your patient comments to life. In most organizations, this is an underutilized resource in making improvements toward patient- and family-centered care.

Patient stories

Beyond a formal structure of a PFAC, there are so many other ways to continually infuse the voices of the patients and families into everything we do. One of the best strategies for this that can be culture-changing for an organization is to start every meeting with a patient story and/or comment. One of the most powerful things I've seen quality committees of the board do is include a patient story that did not go well at the top of their meeting. The idea is that "There's always room for improvement," and "Our work is not done until we have no more stories like this to share." Beyond the bad ones, though, having a mechanism to share patient stories is powerful to caregivers.

When I was in high school, I was often teased by some of my friends when I would tell a story and go on and on with extra details and they'd say, "Point?"

And while it was teenage teasing, I've thought of that over the years and realized that storytelling doesn't come naturally to everyone. Some of us who might think we're good at telling stories may also have room to improve.

There are whole conferences and sessions on how to improve your storytelling. I won't profess to be an expert on this, as I believe we can all continue to grow in our storytelling abilities. Storytelling can be an effective tool to help capture the imagination, engage emotion, and open minds of the listeners. According to the Storytelling Arts of Indiana, "Storytellers are 'directors of the theater of the mind,' co-creating the story's images and emotions with the audience. Sharing stories builds community … from one listener to the next" (n.d.).

I was shadow coaching with a provider who was initially pretty resistant to being coached. (I think his medical director may have even had to promise him dinner at the local steakhouse if this provider didn't learn something from me in the coaching session. Seriously, no pressure there!) Anyway, the provider and I got through our coaching session and were talking about his strengths and opportunities in a debrief session.

This provider turned out to be pretty passionate about patient experience. He harkened back to a workshop that I had facilitated and he had attended where we had shared a video filmed entirely from the patient's viewpoint. This provider talked about how he himself had never been a patient, and how seeing things from that lens made such a difference to him.

That's the reason we share the patient and family stories. When you're doing so, get creative. Finding ways to record video and share those stories is very powerful. When you can't get someone on camera or they're not comfortable with that, there are other ways to be creative. We've also told a story with animated typing where the letters fly in on a black background. The room grows silent, as everyone must read the story—a very powerful and profound way to share a story.

Patient speakers

This may seem obvious to some, but whenever you're having a symposium within the organization—a leadership meeting, a quality team presentation, anything of that nature—strive to have a patient be there to share his or her story. I've seen patient speakers be compelling and important parts of key organizational sessions. This is most effective to help ground teams and leaders ahead of whatever else they are there to discuss.

Looking back at some of the conferences and presentations I've made within organizations over the years, I always strived to start with the voice of the patient—usually by sharing a patient comment or story. However, if I could do it again, I would have worked harder to ensure that we were able to have a patient or family member physically present to share his or her story. Physical presence has an added impact that just can't be captured in the same way by someone else reading the story. In some patient experience departments, there is one main staff person who is most connected with the patient and family members who serve throughout the organization. This person is effective in helping to identify people with a story that would fit for various meetings and topics. And that person can also be adept at helping to prepare the patient and helping him or her tell the story in the most effective way.

Patients serving on committees

When patients are joining healthcare committees for the first time, there are often challenges depending on their ability to communicate and be heard by the healthcare team. While some groups are especially patient, I've seen the healthcare team tune out if a patient story is rambling and goes on too long, or even if it's a great story but the point is not made to help relate to the topic at hand.

One way to combat this is by helping to coach patient and family advisors as to how to tell their story before they serve on committees. By using a

Chapter 4

methodology such as ISBAR, with which most of the care team members are already familiar, this can help patients to tell their stories in a manner that the healthcare team is more readily able to hear.

This is not about trying to change the voices of patients and families. Rather, it's about helping patients and families speak in a language and manner that healthcare providers can understand, so they are more likely to truly hear the main point of that message.

ISBAR

ISBAR (pronounced *eye-s-bar*) is a mnemonic tool used to help standardize communication of critical information to improve safety.

ISBAR stands for:

- I = Identify (State your name, role, position, location)
- S = Situation (State the purpose – "I am calling to … ")
- B = Background (Tell the story of the current problem)
- A = Assessment (State what you think is going on)
- R = Recommendation (What do you recommend or want the person to whom you're talking to do?)

In healthcare, ISBAR is used with clinical handoffs for patients and to provide the opportunity for providers to both ask and respond to key questions from other care team members. It is also used to help facilitate communication within disciplines, including—but certainly not limited to—reports to other team members about a change in patient status, transfers of care, etc.

Many hospitals have instituted ISBAR as part of their standard handoff for all patient-related communications. This is often utilized as a best practice to help meet the Joint Commission National Patient Safety Goal with regards to developing a standardized approach to handoff communications (Agency for Healthcare Research and Quality, 2015).

In the clinical setting, the recommendation is related to the patient's status, so that the most critical information is efficiently shared and is able to result in an acceptable plan of care by both parties.

This method can translate into other aspects of communication as well—even nonclinical. Consider this example for a patient joining a committee and sharing a story:

- I = Identify

    "My name is Janiece, and I was recently a patient in your clinic at the 8100 building."

- S = Situation

    "I want to make you aware about something that happened while I was a patient there."

- B = Background

    "I'd had a cold or respiratory something for about two weeks, and I'd been traveling quite a bit. In my work I am in and out of a lot of hospitals, and I wanted to make sure that whatever I had was not contagious. When I called to make the appointment, I was told to arrive at 8:45, ahead of my 9:00 appointment. I arrived and was roomed right away, but then I waited in the exam room for over an hour. When I finally saw Dr. Peterson, he didn't even acknowledge that he was late or offer any explanation."

- A = Assessment

    "This particular time I had the same experience that I've had repeatedly when seeing this provider. This is not my usual provider, but he seems to be the only one available when I call in for a more urgent

Chapter 4

> appointment. My husband also had this happen earlier this year when he called for an appointment and was scheduled with a different physician."

- R = Recommendation

  "I'd like to suggest that we look at the scheduling for those physicians and see if this is happening to others beyond those I've identified. It would be good to look at the sources of delays for the physicians and and also to talk to the providers about what they see and feel about their schedules. It also would be helpful to offer him some coaching on how to start off a visit when he is running late. A simple word or phrase to acknowledge the wait would have made a big difference to me."

This example is a great way of showing how a patient or family member could share a story in a meaningful and succinct way while still getting the point across with a recommendation to the healthcare team.

Not only is it important to prepare patient and family representatives of committees, but an often missed step when having patients join committees is to remember to prepare team members for hearing patient feedback. This is one of those things that you may not think about until you don't think about it and then get caught in a difficult situation. I've found that it is very easy for staff and physicians to become defensive depending on how and what patients and families are sharing. I always encourage groups that I work with to be open and to try to suspend judgment when they hear the patient's perspectives. Preparing caregivers to truly be ready to hear and listen to the story is important as well. Listening is not just a skill, it's a choice—one that each of us chooses to make (or not) every day.

"When I listen, I have the power. When I speak, I give it away." —Voltaire

Patient fears

Regardless of the state of your patient and family involvement in your organization, there are ample other studies of what patients and families are most concerned about. Whether you are struggling to create a PFAC in your organization, or you find it difficult to engage patients and families in your work, know that there are other ways to also get at patients' and families' wants and needs. I mention this as a resource to you, so if you find yourself in need of insight from patients and families and your PFAC doesn't meet for another two months, or the aspect that you need hasn't been covered, or their upcoming agenda is full, know that there are other sources of information available to you (see the references list for more information).

One of the most formative studies in my work in this area was performed by a dear friend and gifted colleague, Colleen Sweeney. Through her research, titled *The Patient Empathy Project,* she found that 96% of people have some fear regarding healthcare (Webster, 2011).

As part of this work, Colleen interviewed patients about what they fear in hospitals and healthcare systems. She found that the most common patient fears are:

- Infection
- Incompetence
- Death
- Cost
- Mix-ups
- Needles
- Rude doctors and nurses

Chapter 4

- Germs
- Prognosis
- Communication issues
- Loneliness

Knowing what these fears are is huge in meeting patients' needs and alleviating what they are most concerned about. Colleen's work is helpful in understanding the key behaviors that everyone can be mindful of in making a difference in the patient experience. Regardless of the sources of data in your own organization, knowing that these are common fears across all patients is an important factor in designing whatever improvements you seek to create.

"Why don't we ask people what their greatest fear is?" Colleen said. "Part of the reason is that we're afraid to know. We're afraid we can't deal with it. But we need to look the patient in the eyes and find out … find out what the patient needs and then do something about it. That's empathy."

After doing this research, Colleen developed a hierarchy of patient needs (see Figure 4.4) that, if met, will help to deliver on the "exceptional patient experience" (2016).

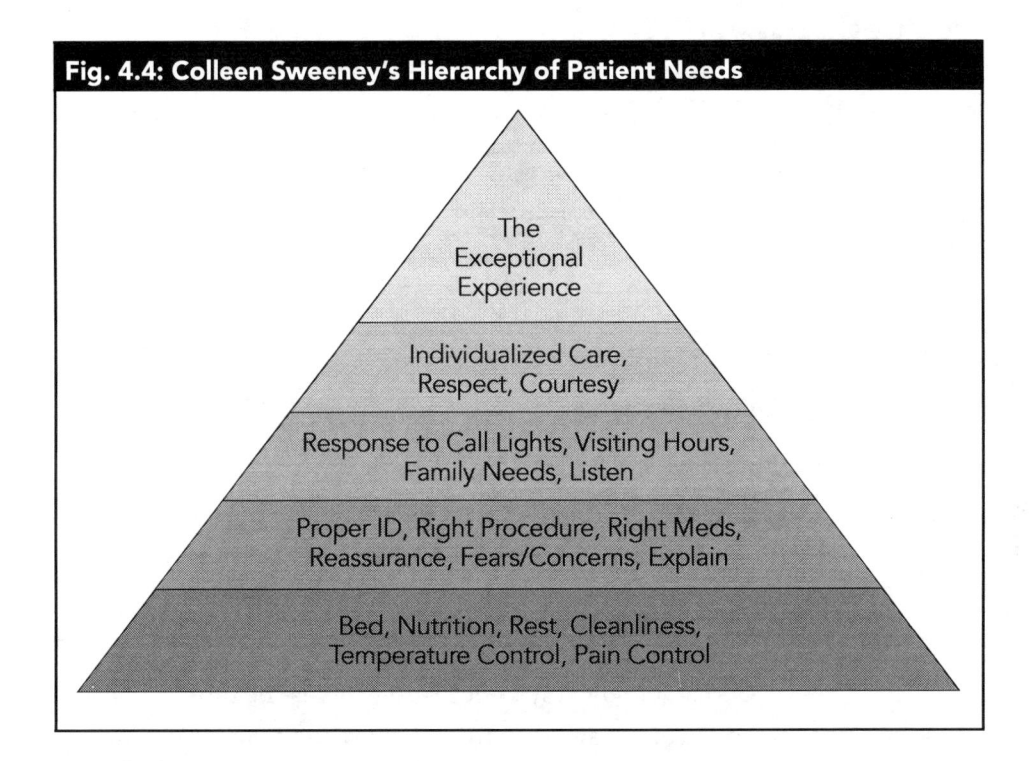

Fig. 4.4: Colleen Sweeney's Hierarchy of Patient Needs

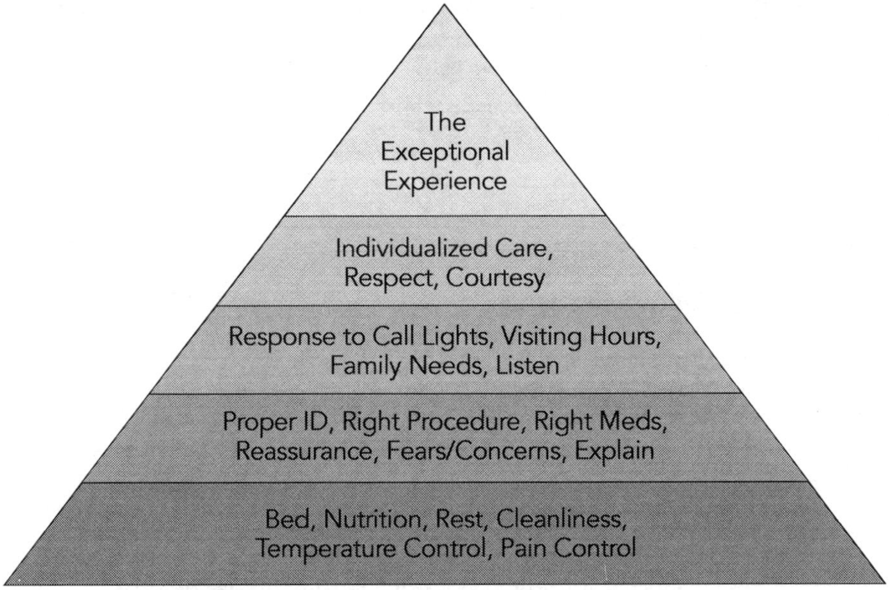
The Exceptional Experience
Individualized Care, Respect, Courtesy
Response to Call Lights, Visiting Hours, Family Needs, Listen
Proper ID, Right Procedure, Right Meds, Reassurance, Fears/Concerns, Explain
Bed, Nutrition, Rest, Cleanliness, Temperature Control, Pain Control

What makes waiting hard

Building on Colleen Sweeney's work in patient fears, another of my favorite authors is David Maister with his work on what makes waiting so difficult. Think about how much waiting there is in healthcare:

- Waiting to be seen in the emergency room
- Waiting for an appointment with a specialist
- Waiting for test results from a breast biopsy
- Waiting for a room to open up in an assisted living facility
- Waiting for a call-back from a pediatrician
- Waiting for someone to answer a call light
- Waiting for an overdue baby to be born

Chapter 4

- Waiting for the medical equipment to come
- Waiting for a family member to pass

The list could go on and on because waiting, in some form or fashion, is embedded into the journey for every patient and family member. In his work, *The Psychology of Waiting Lines,* Maister describes how waiting is harder when:

- The wait time is unknown
- The waiting is unexplained
- The waiting seems unfair
- Your time is unoccupied time (distractions)
- You are anxious
- You are alone (1985)

This feels like a checklist for so many of our care settings. Be mindful of these concerns and strategize how to address them with proactive communication, frequent updates, distractions/amenities, and personal presence. Incorporating these will not only make a difference in the lives of your patients and families, but it can also help to reduce frustration on the part of the care team.

Listening to your patients and families and projecting their voices into your organization is a great strategy to help engage the physicians and staff with your efforts. We've reviewed several key ways to involve patients and families in your work. We've suggested ways to harness their voices through what they are already telling you (i.e., comments and complaints) and create structures for them to speak into (e.g., PFACs, serving on committees). We also reviewed some resources about what's most important to patients, their fears, and their concerns from which you can draw on while formalizing your own mechanisms for obtaining patient feedback. Establishing common ground with the care team by having the initial focus on the patient is a great way to orient your work for improvement. While an important starting point, this is by no means the end point of your improvement journey. Next up: a focus on the people who provide the care to your patients and families.

References

Agency for Healthcare Research and Quality. (2015). Handoffs and signouts. Retrieved June 27, 2016, from *https://psnet.ahrq.gov/primers/primer/9/handoffs-and-signouts*

Department for Health and Ageing, Government of South Australia. (2016). ISBAR: A standard mnemonic to improve clinical communication. *SA Health.* Retrieved June 27, 2016, from *http://goo.gl/DhtKMu*

Fagan, M., Wong, C., & Carnie, M. (2015). *Brigham and Women's Hospital Patient and Family Advisory Council (PFAC) Report.* Brigham and Women's Hospital. Retrieved June 27, 2016, from *www.ipfcc.org/advance/topics/annual-report-bwhc-2015.pdf*

Landro, L. (2013). More hospitals use social media to gather feedback from patients' families. *The Wall Street Journal.* Retrieved June 27, 2016, from *www.wsj.com/articles/SB10001424127887324108204579022843109511438*

Maister, D. (1985). The psychology of waiting lines. In J. A. Czepiel, M. R. Solomon, and C.F. Surprenant (Eds.), *The Service encounter: Managing employee/customer interaction in service businesses.* Lexington, MA: D. C. Heath and Company, Lexington Books.

Meghan West and Laurie Brown Skunks Team. (n.d.) Patient and Family Advisory Council—Getting Started Tool Kit. BJC HealthCare. Retrieved June 27, 2016, from *http://c.ymcdn.com/sites/www.theberylinstitute.org/resource/resmgr/webinar_pdf/pfac_toolkit_shared_version.pdf*

Storytelling Arts of Indiana. (n.d.). Reviews and resources. Retrieved June 27, 2016, from *http://storytellingarts.org/resources/*

Van de Ven, A. H. (2014) What matters most to patients? Participative provider care and staff courtesy. *Patient Experience Journal,* (1)1, Article 17. Retrieved June 27, 2016, from *http://pxjournal.org/cgi/viewcontent.cgi?article=1004&context=journal*

Rodak, S. (2012). Very important factors contributing to patients' healthcare experience. *Becker's Hospital Review.* Retrieved June 27, 2016, from *www.beckershospitalreview.com/strategic-planning/report-10-qvery-importantq-factors-contributing-to-patients-healthcare-experience.html*

Rickert, J. (2012). Patient-centered care: What it means and how to get there. Retrieved June 27, 2016, from *http://healthaffairs.org/blog/2012/01/24/patient-centered-care-what-it-means-and-how-to-get-there/*

Sweeney, C. (2016). The patient empathy project: Dealing with patient fears improves experience. NetworkNews. Retrieved June 27, 2016, from *https://hartfordhealthcare.org/ File%20Library/Publications/Network%20News/NetworkNews-Feb-2016.pdf*

The Beryl Institute. (2012). Retrieved from *http://c.ymcdn.com/sites/www.the beryl institute.org/resource/resmgr/Conference_2012/Beryl_Keynote_Presentation_f.pdf?hh SearchTerms=%22empathy+and+project%22*

Webster, A. (2011). Easing patient fears can raise HCAHPS scores. HealthLeaders Media. Retrieved June 27, 2016, from *www.healthleadersmedia.com/marketing/ easing-patient-fears-can-raise-hcahps-scores*

Chapter 5
People Are the Reason We Excel

"Patients are the reason we exist; people are the reason we excel."

The president of the hospital where I had my first job out of grad school strongly believed this, and he shared it repeatedly with his staff. I had no idea at that point so early in my career that those words would stick with me. But they really turned out to be formative to my approach and philosophy of management and leadership.

Even now, in the work that I do with frontline staff groups and with leaders, I draw back on that philosophy. It's a great approach to keep us all grounded in the simple fact that if there were no patients, we wouldn't have jobs. And yet, the only way we can truly provide for the patients who entrust us with their care is if we enable the people on our teams to excel in their roles.

In the last chapter we talked about connection and how the voices of the patients are one of the best ways to engage caregivers. Understanding the importance of connection from a staff perspective and their engagement is also crucial to success.

When I am working with teams of frontline staff, there's usually at least one person who says, "I'm not here to talk about the patient experience; I want to talk about *my* experience as a staff member in this department." Leaders who don't listen, acknowledge, and address these types of concerns won't be able to realize their patient experience goals. Often, it's not major issues that are holding the staff back from wanting to participate in improving the care they provide; rather, they are issues that are very much able to be addressed.

I was talking with a patient experience director recently about the work she was doing in a clinic with a busy front desk area. The staff members spent a lot of time on the phone answering calls and booking appointments, as well as greeting patients as they arrived. The patient experience director was talking to them about being a better listener and how that was one of the focus areas for that clinic, as they'd seen some of their scores dip. The team member looked at the director and said, "Well, if you can fix this dang fan in the ceiling over my head, I surely will be able to do a better job of listening because I'll be able to actually *hear* my patients!"

This director went on to talk about how in that clinic they had gone on to identify a host of environmental and process issues that were prohibiting staff from providing the best care possible to their patients. She said, "These are all real, important, and not that expensive to fix!"

Bottom line: It is essential to connect and not only hear but truly listen to the teams providing the care to make a difference in the overall patient experience and environment of care. I've seen too many leaders (including patient experience leaders) railroad through a team and not stop to listen to the true concerns from the staff. When we bulldoze over the concerns in this manner and do so in the name of patient experience, it makes the work before us that much more difficult.

In his book *Patients Come Second*, Paul Spiegelman writes: "In any business, you can't take care of customers if you don't take care of employees. Healthcare is no different. We must find ways to engage our nurses, administrative staff, physicians, housekeeping staff, supervisors, switchboard operators, etc., so that they WANT to provide great service to their patients. It's not that we think patients are not important. But there is a direct correlation between employee loyalty and customer loyalty" (2013).

The sooner we can embrace this reality and start to focus on the needs of our employees and to let them *know* that, the sooner we'll be able to make improvements in the care and the culture of the organization.

The exciting part is that organizations are starting to make this connection between patient experience and employee engagement. In the past year alone, I've been a part of three projects that started out as a patient experience/service culture improvement project, but then the organization stepped back, refocused, and embarked instead on an employee engagement/engaged culture project. In each of these organizations, improving their patient experience and truly achieving patient- and family-centered care was still at the heart of their efforts, but they realized they couldn't do patient experience justice without focusing on their staff and physicians first.

Connection Between Employee Engagement and Patient Experience

It's not just happenstance that these organizations are choosing to focus on their employees first. There's more than ample support for the notion that staff engagement directly contributes to a positive patient experience.

According to a 2013 article in the *Harvard Business Review*, "Engaging those employees around the behaviors and skills that drive clinical excellence and a positive patient experience is going to be a key factor in determining whether a hospital thrives—or even survives—in this new environment." This is a bit of a challenge when the Willis Towers Watson's most recent global workforce study found that less than half (44%) of the U.S. hospital workforce overall is highly engaged. Their *2012 Global Workforce Study* provides insight into the attitudes and concerns of 32,000 workers around the world and across various industries. Some of the highlights include:

- Stress and anxiety about the future are common

- Job security takes precedence over almost everything

- Attracting employees is almost entirely about security, while retaining employees has more to do with the quality of the work experience overall

- Employees have doubts about the level of interest and support coming from senior leaders

Willis Towers Watson also performed a regression analysis of their findings and examined key drivers of an engaging work experience, specifically within the healthcare industry.

Fig. 5.1: Willis Towers Watson Drivers of Engagement

Drivers of Engagement in the U.S. Healthcare Industry

LEADERSHIP	STRESS, BALANCE AND WORKLOAD
Is effective at growing the business	Stress levels at work are manageable
Shows sincere interest in employees' well-being	There is a healthy balance between work and personal life
Behaves consistently with the organization's care values	Work arrangements are flexible
Demonstrates trust and confidence in the job being done	Work groups have adequate staff to do the job

GOAL AND OBJECTIVES	CAREER DEVELOPMENT
Employees understand the organization's business goals and steps needed to reach them	Employees have opportunities for personal development and advancement
Employees understand how their jobs contribute to the organization achieving its goals	Organization provides career planning tools, resources, and training

SUPERVISION	
Managers treat staff with respect	Managers act in ways consistent with their words
They encourage new ideas and ways of doing things	They lead effective career development conversations

Source: Willis Towers Watson

Summarized broadly, teamwork, empowerment, and career advancement opportunities are some of the greatest predictors of employee engagement. There are some very tangible takeaways for leaders and organizations in terms of actionable behaviors and activities to help promote greater employee engagement.

My approach, when assessing an organization's culture and helping to develop a strategy for success, is to consider not only their patient experience data but also their employee engagement, physician satisfaction (if they have it), and even safety culture survey data. These combined sources really help to give an in-depth picture of the organization. The connection between these aspects and patient experience improvement has been well documented.

Most recently, patient experience was associated with more favorable clinical outcomes. Trzeciak et al, found "statistically significant association between patient experience star ratings and multiple clinical outcomes, with the most consistent associations found between a higher number of stars for patient experience and lower rates of readmission to the hospital" (2016). (See the reference list for more information.)

Connecting People to Purpose

One of the best ways to truly engage staff and physicians is to reconnect them with why they got into the jobs and roles that they chose. I can assure you that 90% of them did so because they wanted to make a difference and help people. Yes, there are the other 10% that are in it for the prestige, the money, and the benefits, whatever. When I teach classes and speak to physicians and staff, I often use this premise of "helping others" to start and reground them in the purpose. So much of the work in changing the culture of the organization revolves around employees and physicians reaffirming their purpose and why they do what they do. For many of them, really for most of them, the healthcare environment in which they pledged to make a difference has changed. In fact, it has changed so dramatically that, for some of them, if they were honest, they may not still choose to do this work in this environment if they were starting out today. Consider the impacts that have come about in just the past 15 years (Saver, 2006):

- The proliferation of electronic medical records
- Nursing shortages
- Huge advancements in medical technology
- Significant transition from fee-for-service to value-based payment
- Consolidation of independent practices and hospitals into large systems
- An aging population and a rise in chronically ill and higher-acuity patients

Given these enormous changes affecting our physicians and nurses, it's no wonder that they are scratching their heads and wondering if they still want to be here. Many will cite the number of hours spent in front of a computer versus a patient, the large amount of documentation, or the myriad forms and paperwork required just to provide the care that they do as issues that affect their work. It is important to give people the space to reflect on why they signed up to do what they do and to assess why they still sign up for it when they walk through the doors for each new shift.

It's only right that we pause and invite our staff and physicians to consider if they will truly recommit to the profession and to the organization that they have chosen. It's only fair that we allow and invite this in our organizations, even if it is a scary conversation. Many leaders worry, "What if they all leave?" The reality is that they won't all leave, but the approach is important if we want to have the right people engaged in the right work in the organization. (See the reference list for more information.)

Active Listening

One activity that I've used in a group setting to help caregivers reconnect with why they entered the field is to do an active listening exercise. Here's the how-to:

- Divide the group into pairs and either have them sit facing each other, or (I think it's even more effective) have them sit facing opposite directions but with their shoulders aligned.

- Have each pair determine who will be the first to talk and who will be the first to listen.

- The talker must talk for the entire time (usually 90 seconds to 2 minutes).

- The listener must listen and not say anything during that time.

- Give them some questions to discuss and share about. I'd suggest something like "Why are you here? How did you get here? Why do you stay here [in this role, this organization]?"
- When the talker is done talking, the listener must then repeat back to them the main points of what they heard (give them about 30 seconds to do so).
- Then they switch roles and do it again.

This activity is helpful to reconnect the care team members with their sense of purpose and why they came into the medical field but also reconnect them with the organization and why they choose to stay here. Furthermore, it's an excellent activity to see what it feels like to be truly listened to, without interruption, and also what it's like to truly listen to another person.

Frontline Example

Recently I was in a conversation with a very fired-up and passionate nurse who works in a busy emergency department in a large suburb of the Twin Cities in Minnesota. This person was talking about the multitude of changes that she'd experienced in her 11 years of working there. She talked about how the culture had changed over time as it related to improvement and accountability. There was a point a few years back where she didn't want to get involved with improvement efforts of any kind within the department. The reason was there was a group of "bullies" as she called them—people who were set in their ways and unwilling to change—who sabotaged any improvement efforts brought forward. She herself stepped back from a charge nurse role and any other leadership activities at that time.

Then there were some positive changes in leadership; new leaders came who set a vision and started to hold people accountable. This led to some significant turnover in the department, but, as she told me, "It was healthy turnover. We had a lot of people leave during that time. But now, some of the good ones who left before all of that are starting to come back." At this point with the changes she's seeing, this nurse is now starting to get back into some of that improvement work and is really excited about the possibilities to set a new course for the culture of the department.

An Engaged Culture … You Can Feel It

Recently, I was able to experience an engaged culture, and it was where I was least expecting it: North Junior High. I was attending a parent "step-up" night for my soon-to-be seventh grader. My husband was out of town, I was running late, I hadn't had dinner, and naturally I got there at 6:05 p.m. as the presentation was already in session. I was not really looking forward to the evening. I expected a bunch of forms, some boring lectures, and let's face it: I was not too keen on the idea of my baby going to junior high.

As I entered the cafeteria, lining the side of the room were all of these people standing. "Shoot, it's standing room only!" I thought. But I quickly noticed plenty of open seats were available. Despite my personal chaos, I was able to note the energy in the room. I sat down and soon realized that the 40-some people lining the side of the room were many of the teachers, staying late after a long day to be there for this session. As the principal talked, I was again amazed at the vibe in the room. This continued throughout the evening.

In the last classroom I visited, I sat in a circle with several other first-time junior high parents, and we met with one of the teachers for next year. One parent asked, "What advice do you have for us as parents?" The teacher saw right through our anxiety (and our held-back tears) and said, "You need to know that everyone in this building is teaching in the grade that they want to in the school that they want to be in. We are a terrifically engaged team and we want to be here to work with your children." I can't tell you how reassuring that was to us as parents, and suddenly most (not all) of my anxiety about my daughter going to this big school, growing up, and making this transition, subsided.

Chapter 5

The event ended at 7:30 p.m., and at 7:35 I made my way to the band room. I talked to the band director and looked around a bit. As I left, I thanked him for being there. With a cheerful smile he shot back, "Thank *you* for being here!" I told this story to my daughter when I got home and couldn't believe that there was a group of teachers who all needed to be back at school in less than 12 hours, calmly and patiently answering our questions.

When I shared this with my husband later that night he teased me saying, "Boy, they sure sold you!" I realized I had met all of these teachers for just a few moments, but you know what? I believed them. That's what an engaged culture can be—you can feel it. I felt it the minute I opened the door to the cafeteria, and I saw it throughout the rest of the evening.

That's what we're striving for on behalf of our patients and families: an engaged culture that they can *feel*. What blows them away is when they aren't expecting it. And it can have the greatest impact on them when they need it most. I went to my daughter's school expecting a bunch of forms and boredom, and instead, I felt nurtured and cared for as some of my worries were shared, reassured, and alleviated.

Building a Culture

> "A person who feels appreciated will always do more than what is expected."
>
> —Author unknown

One of the easiest things that leaders can do is to see and acknowledge the great work of their staff. I'm a huge believer in the power of positive coaching and will devote an entire chapter to it later on. In my experience coaching hundreds of physicians, nurses, and techs all around the country, I've learned that people are craving some affirmation. They don't walk around looking needy, but they blossom when we give them some positive feedback.

People Are the Reason We Excel

The same leader who taught me the "Patients are the reason we exist; people are the reason we excel" mantra also instilled in me the value of thanking people. This person strived to write at least five thank-you notes each week. I took that to heart and tried to incorporate that throughout my roles over time. I'm not very good about being consistent, but I do try to incorporate this and send handwritten thank-you notes as much as possible. Email is great, but sending a personal note or card still gets noticed.

Finding ways to instill into leaders, staff, and physicians the value of thanking and appreciating one another is a tremendous way to change the culture. Most organizations have a currency by which they do this. For some it's "UR Remarkable" cards, or a "Kudos" card, or a "Wow" card, or just a "Thank You" card. Many of them are available to staff, leaders, and patients. Usually, when they are turned in, they are shared with the staff member's manager and then given to the team member themselves. For some organizations, these cards can be redeemed in the gift shop or other places in the building.

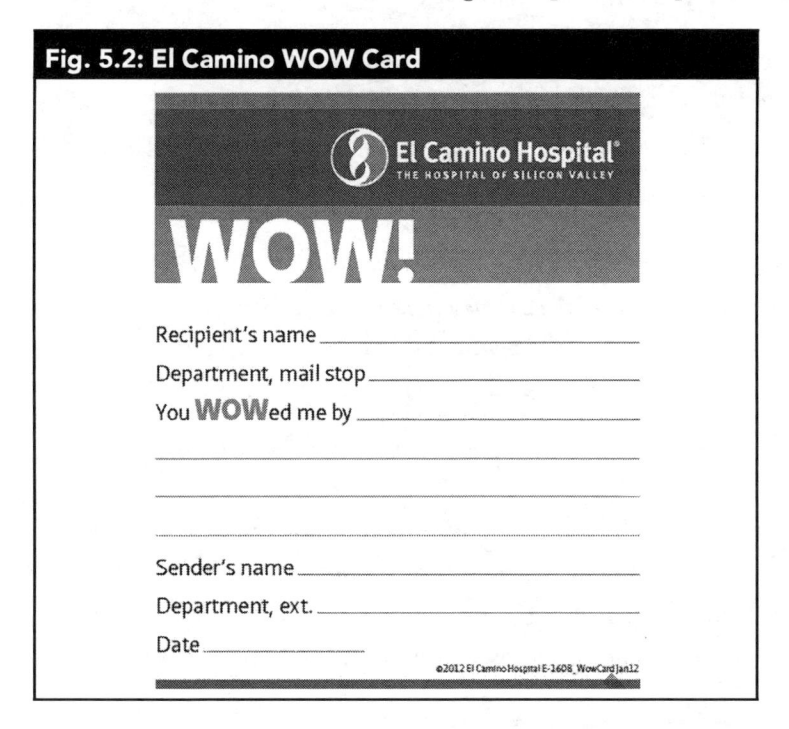

Fig. 5.2: El Camino WOW Card

Chapter 5

In one organization, while talking about the value of thanking, we came across a story told to us by one staff member about a scene he'd witnessed in his department. For whatever the reason, he'd never felt comfortable sharing it with those involved, so anonymously he shared this with us. The room was silent as the text appeared on the screen and people read it to themselves:

> *A patient was coming from the care center and had no family here and was dying, so the nurse went out to find someone to take her other patients.*
>
> *Then she sat in the room, closed the door, turned the light down, held the patient's hand, and sat with her while the patient was passing on.*
>
> *She just kept reassuring the patient that she wasn't alone. The nurse wanted the family to know that the patient wasn't alone when she had passed away.*
>
> *The other part of it is that there was another nurse.*
>
> *The one who stepped up and took care of the other patients, adding more to her assignment to enable the other nurse to be able to be with the patient.*
>
> *It was really well done.*
>
> *In this busy department for something of that magnitude to happen, it's tough, but they made it happen. They made it work because for that patient, it was the moment that the patient was passing on—there is no opportune time.*
>
> *Nicely done for both nurses. That's good service, good care, kindness.*

We shared this at an empathy workshop and then handed out the organization's thank-you cards and gave each person an opportunity to write one. We encouraged them to think about their last shift, their last week, their last month, and identify someone who came to mind who they saw in action and never got a chance to truly stop and tell them in the moment how much they appreciated what they did. This could be something that was done for another staff person or something that they did for a patient.

After one of these workshops with the night shift, I was coaching one of the social workers who had attended. One of the things I affirmed as her strength was her thanking of others and her patients. She got this sly smile and said, "Well, I just have to tell you. After that workshop the other night, a group of us went to work and throughout the entire shift we were being sarcastic smart alecs"—my word, not hers—"and *overthanking* each other. 'Oh, thank you,' 'No, thank *you*' for the silliest stuff. But then, all of a sudden we witnessed someone do something amazing for one of our patients and we all said, 'We need to find one of those dang cards—we need to thank her!' "

I share this story because I love that even in their silliness they were able to learn something, and that it stuck with them. When you have ignited or reignited a culture that sees the value, and feels the permission and the responsibility to thank one another in the care that they provide, it can truly help to make a lasting difference.

We've talked about various reasons to incorporate employee engagement efforts into your patient experience strategy. Beyond that, we've explored some strategies for how to reconnect and engage physicians and staff with this work. It's imperative to be mindful of these aspects when seeking this type of improvement in your organization.

References

Anderson, A. (2014). The impact of the Affordable Care Act on the health care workforce. Retrieved June 27, 2016, from *www.heritage.org/research/reports/2014/03/ the-impact-of-the-affordable-care-act-on-the-health-care-workforce*

Peltier, J., and Dahl, A. (2009). The relationship between employee satisfaction and hospital patient experiences. Retrieved June 27, 2016, from *www.info-now.com/typo3conf/ ext/p2wlib/pi1/press2web/html/userimg/FORUM/Hospital%20Study%20-Relationship%20 Btwn%20Emp.%20Satisfaction%20and%20Pt.%20Experiences.pdf*

Saver, C. L. (2006). Nursing—today and beyond. Retrieved June 27, 2016, from *https://americannursetoday.com/nursing-today-and-beyond/*

Sherwood, R. (2013). Employee engagement drives health care quality and financial returns. Retrieved June 27, 2016, from *https://hbr.org/2013/10/employee-engagement-drives-health-care-quality-and-financial-returns*

Spiegelman, P., and Berrett, B. (2013). *Patients Come Second.* Windsor, CT: The Donohue Group, Inc. Retrieved: *http://patientscomesecond.com/*

The Beryl Institute. (n.d.). Patient experience case study—Elmhurst. Retrieved June 27, 2016, from *www.theberylinstitute.org/default.asp?page=CASE0912*

Tiffin, C. (2012). Beyond the bedside: The changing role of today's nurses. Retrieved June 27, 2016, from *www.huffingtonpost.com/charles-tiffin-phd/nursing-school_b_1384285.html*

Trzeciak, S., Gaughan, J. P, Bosire, J., and Mazzarelli, A. J. (2016). Association between Medicare summary star ratings for patient experience and clinical outcomes in US hospitals. *Journal of Patient Experience,* 3(1) 6–9.

Willis Towers Watson. (2014). *The 2014 Global Workforce Study.* Retrieved June 27, 2016, from *www.towerswatson.com/en-US/Insights/IC-Types/Survey-Research-Results/2014/08/the-2014-global-workforce-study*

Willis Towers Watson. (2012). *The 2012 Global Workforce Study.* Retrieved June 27, 2016, from *www.towerswatson.com/en/Insights/IC-Types/Survey-Research-Results/2012/07/2012-Towers-Watson-Global-Workforce-Study*

Willis Towers Watson. (2010). Case Study: A large hospital network links employee engagement with patient satisfaction to maximize competitive strength. Retrieved June 27, 2016, from *www.towerswatson.com/en-US/Insights/IC-Types/Case-Studies/2010/Case-Study-A-Large-Hospital-Network-Links-Employee-Engagement-with-Patient-Satisfaction-to-Maximiz*

Section 3
Structure

Chapter 6
Setting Up for Success

We've started with a focus and understanding of the compulsories and spent time looking at the means of connection for staff and physicians: projecting the voices of patients and also focusing on engagement strategies. As we start to talk about collaboration, we need to look at how to work across the organization creating focused improvements. To do this, it's important to look at how best to structure resources within the organization to support the work. This may sound easy, but there are so many factors to consider. Finding the right people for the right roles, including finding the right executive sponsors, is no small feat. Since this is such a passion of mine, patient experience, I sometimes find it hard and have to remember that it's not everyone else's passion.

The field of patient experience professionals is growing. It's so much more robust now, with so many more options for support and resources than it had when I started in it eight-plus years ago. Organizations like the Beryl Institute and Institute for Patient- and Family-Centered Care have so much to offer organizations and individuals working in this area. At this point, most organizations have committed to making improvements and realize they need some level of resources to do so. In this section, we'll look at some considerations for organizations as they set up their structure.

Chapter 6

Scope

One of the first considerations from a sponsorship, steering team oversight, and frontline improvement leadership perspective includes the scope. Are we looking across the continuum focused on hospitals, clinics, home health, long-term care, emergency departments, and ambulatory surgery? For many organizations, this scope is huge. In others, they choose to deploy the resources to certain areas. This may include just the hospital with a core focus on Hospital Consumer Assessment of Healthcare Providers and Systems (HCAHPS) improvement. Or it may be in the clinic with focused improvements in the ambulatory sector.

Whatever the chosen scope, know that there will always be a propensity for scope creep. That's not just a consulting term, but something that I see happen all the time in organizations. One of the reasons I think it's so easy to do with this work is that almost anything and everything can be tied to patient experience. Therefore, the workload and areas of responsibility for the leaders of this area can often morph.

At one point in my career, I was looking at moving to a position within a large hospital for a newly created director of patient experience. Since this was a new position for the organization, they were working with Human Resources to create the job description and skill sets, etc. When we started talks, it made a lot of sense, but by the time I eventually declined the position, it then included a host of other areas including the international medicine program and several other aspects that would have taken a lot of time from the improvement work and focus on patient experience. I jokingly was able to tell the hospital president that since it now included "everything but the kitchen sink," I really didn't think I could be successful in delivering on everything he and I wanted to achieve with this position.

This is all too often the case. The organization knows that it needs a position or someone to be boots-on-the-ground leading this work. And yet, getting the resources to support this position and the focus required and desired is often really hard to do. It's rare that positions are fully dedicated to this work. More often, I see a lot of the "combo platter" positions, where the person is designated with patient experience but it's one of many foods on their plate. This is why it's imperative that the organization has a definition for their patient experience or patient- and family-centered care and know what they are trying to accomplish. Organizations that are able to do this have a better chance of dedicating the resources they need and realizing the success they desire in the parts of the organization where they are focused.

Setting Up For Success: Do You Need a CXO?

I don't usually talk to recruiters, but for some reason, on one particular Monday morning, I did. It was for a CXO (chief experience officer) position at a health system in central Pennsylvania, where I was raised and still have extended family. I told myself it was for the networking … people are always asking us about job opportunities. If I'm truthful, it may have been more to just see what I'm worth out on the open market. I left a gig like that at a large system here in Minnesota a few years ago. Together with a few trusted souls, I helped found DTA Associates, Inc., for the chance to work with healthcare systems throughout the country; I felt no real need to look. However, you always wonder what the job market is out there. So, I talked to her.

Jennifer, the recruiter, was very nice and shared with me a bit about how they are really seeing this as a "trending position" in the market. As we chatted, she shared some of the key categories of people that apply and yet the struggles that they have in finding the truly right fit. Most of the candidates come out of a few areas: hospitality (but limited healthcare exposure), healthcare operations and/or performance improvement (but limited patient experience exposure), or true patient experience background but at a small hospital

Chapter 6

(without demonstrated success across a large system). I quickly saw why she had reached out, as not only did I have the demonstrated patient experience background in a large health system but I also had a clinical social work experience, as well as performance improvement skills. As she said, "the people like you are few and far between."

Many organizations, like the one that Jennifer was recruiting for, are making large investments. In this case they were looking to invest $1 million in patient experience. Of that $1 million–type of investment, a CXO position may be in the range of $250,000 (Barnet, 2015). That's interesting when you think of the dollars at stake in a typical organization's value-based purchasing component. This new role is great for large hospitals and healthcare systems like the one Jennifer was recruiting for that Monday. What about the mid-sized community hospitals? With budgets and people power already stretched, how can those organizations afford these positions? And how can they afford not to?

The role of the CXO is certainly emerging. One of the best descriptions of this was from Donna Padilla of executive search firm Witt/Kieffer, who noted, "It is critical that organizations have a place, and person, at which the buck stops—someone who can not only make sure the valet is opening doors correctly but also, for example, establish metrics, gather data, determine successes and failures, and communicate suggested courses for improvement to the CEO and top administrators" (2014). Jason Wolf and Dan Prince also published some work on the role of the CXO, identifying that it "brings focus to an organization's stated commitment to providing a great patient experience. It offers the potential to align various initiatives and processes around the customer ... it ensures a seat at the table for the voice of the customer to be heard and acted on when senior leaders gather and make decisions" (2014).

That being said, not every organization has or can support the role of a CXO, so in this section we will cover a few types of models that can make a big difference to organizations as they consider what type of internal support structure fits for their organization. Regardless of the model chosen, what's most important is someone who is that "buck stops here" contact related to patient experience.

Internal Support Structure

It's at this point that I need to acknowledge a bias I have about this: I'm not big into building fiefdoms. What I have to say may not be popular to some in the profession of patient experience. I mentioned that at one time I had a department of six devoted to leading patient experience across a huge system. There was some movement at that time, in particular by a physician who had come from another system, to create the Office of Patient Experience. At the time, I couldn't quite articulate why, but I rebelled against that idea. If I'd wanted to, I'm sure I could have worked with this physician to create the office and also negotiate to be the CXO, but that's not what I wanted for myself or for the organization at that point.

Looking back five years later, I can see why I didn't want that and why that philosophically just didn't sit well with me. I strongly advocate that the efforts in patient experience be linked to the efforts in other aspects of safety and quality. The more that patient experience is set aside and held out as this special department, the less integrated it will be with other efforts in the organization. Perhaps the bigger motivation is that I have seen too many highly resourced, set apart departments struggle to maintain their resourcing over time. When patient experience becomes the flavor of last year, then there is vulnerability for these resources within the organization.

Designated or dedicated

One of the first considerations about resourcing leadership in patient experience is whether or not the team/leader is designated or dedicated to work on patient experience improvement. I know this one really sounds like an issue

Chapter 6

of semantics, but it's not! Dedicated is when this is their full-time job and their focus is within patient experience. Designated is when the responsibility for patient experience has been delegated to this person on top of the rest of their already-full plate. "Lucky you, you're now going to lead our patient experience efforts, too!"

I first learned this distinction when working with a large organization that was trying to figure out their structural model. The executive sponsor for patient experience was asked to bring forward a proposal of how she would structure for success in quickly reaching the 90th percentile. (Yep, you can go ahead and chuckle about the *quickly* and *90th percentile* in the same sentence!) She proposed one main patient experience leader at the corporate position, and then a dedicated patient experience team member at each of the local hospitals. For this organization, the structure that she proposed was nearly $1 million annually! You may already be able to guess what happened. Instead of dedicated resources at each of the local organizations, she was asked to designate people to lead patient experience at each of those local sites, in addition to their regular jobs.

Depending on the size of the organization and the timing of where they are at in their improvement journey, one is not necessarily better than another. The obvious considerations are availability of funding and pace and timing of desired improvements. What I tend to recommend is a hybrid model. Even when you have a dedicated team of people, patient experience is truly everyone's responsibility. The challenge is to help make that the focus for the organization. Additionally, it's impossible for one person or even one team to be absolutely everywhere across the organization, so it's important to have local reinforcements. Here are a few ideas of what this can look like in both smaller and larger organizations.

Fig. 6.1: Patient Experience Team Model Hospital

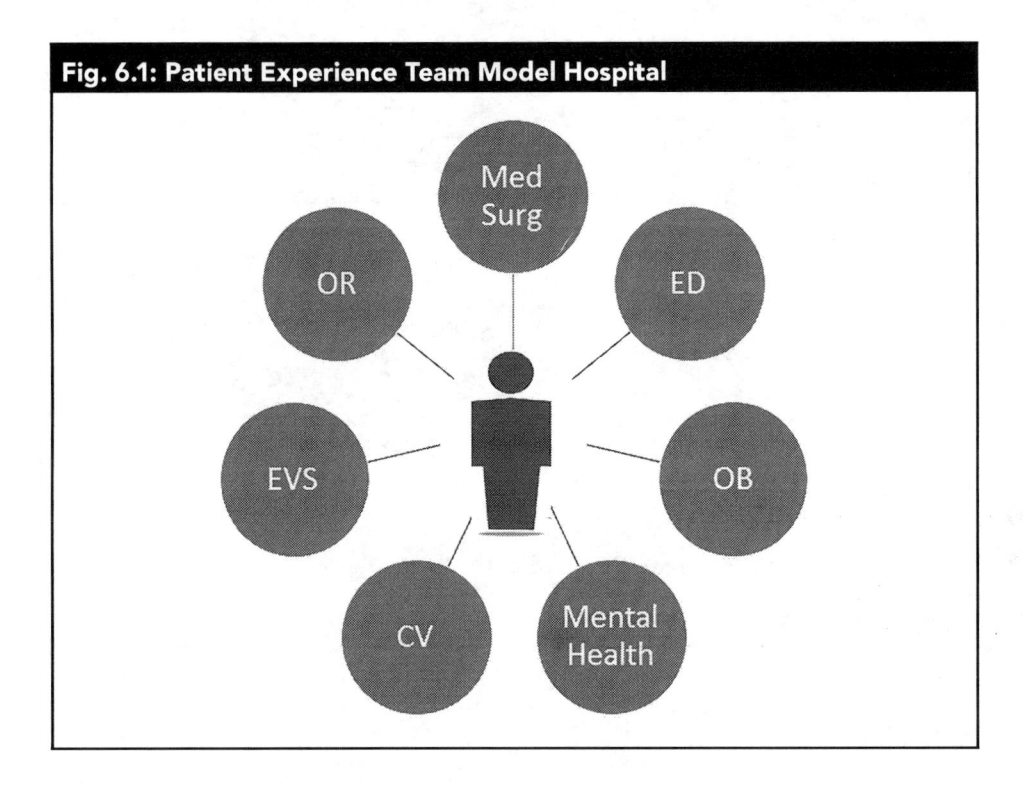

Chapter 6

Fig. 6.2: Patient Experience Team Model System

[Diagram showing central patient experience team connected to: Home Health, Hospital A, Hospital B, Hospital C, Ambulance, Hospice, Clinics, Outpatient Surgery]

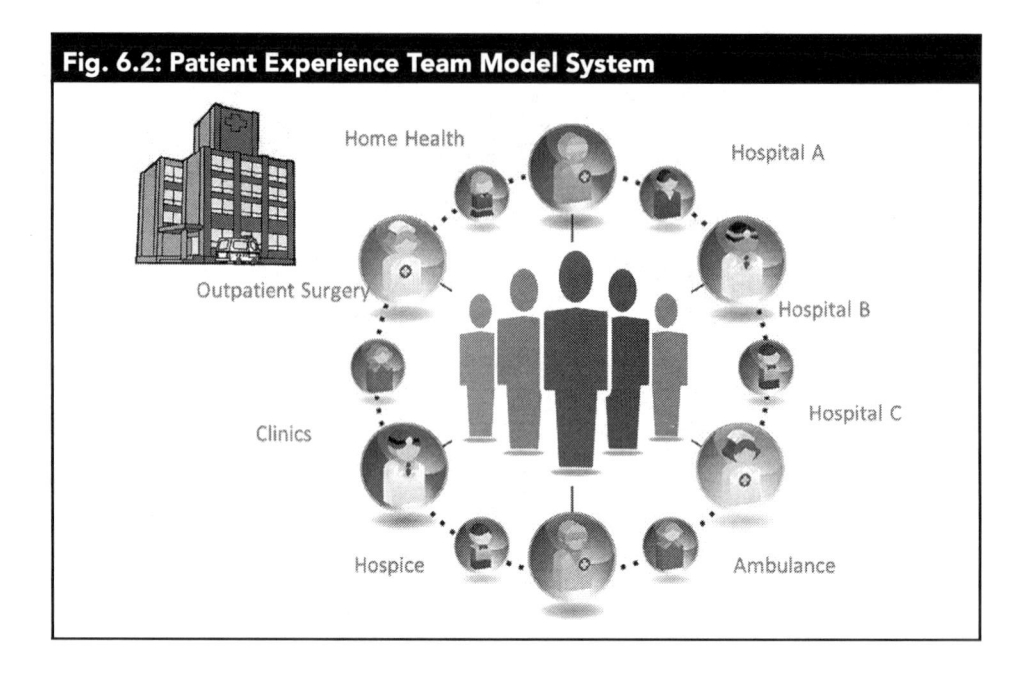

Central vs. local

This discussion leads to an important concept to name, especially for larger organizations. There is this aspect of central vs. local both in terms of resourcing and also in terms of decision and discretion. In working in and with organizations across the country, there is very often this corporate vs. site dynamic.

From a site perspective I've heard: "Well, corporate tells us that we have to focus on bedside shift report, but we've done that here for years and years, and we have our own version and way that it works for us."

From the corporate perspective I've heard: "We're trying to create some similar patient experiences for our patients across the system, so that whether they're a patient in any of our campuses, they'll have some things they can count on that are done the same. Each site seems to want to do their own thing."

Balancing this dynamic from a corporate or central system agenda and a local or site perspective is difficult. I have lived on both sides of that equation, and neither one is particularly easy. Both perspectives are truly valid. The challenge is for the right patient experience leader to balance them both, creating relevant, helpful support for the local units while balancing a systemwide approach to sustained improvements.

My bias is toward having the corporate teams/resources be out at the sites and as connected and visible with them as possible. In most systems there is a perception (somewhat negative) about the corporate teams being less in touch with what's going on at the local levels. When I have led teams with multiple sites (even in smaller organizations), I always encourage/require that we get out and connect with the local sites as much as possible.

One helpful activity for this is a calendar study. I did this once with a patient experience team. We looked at a given week and printed out our outlook calendars, and then looked through and classified our time. We looked at how much time we spent:

- With patients
- With frontline staff
- With physicians
- Engaged in improvement efforts
- Looking at/using our patient experience data (various sources)
- As a team
- In other meetings
- Doing administrative or other tasks

Chapter 6

We did this as a current state assessment just to see where we were spending our time. It was helpful to do this as a team and then look at our aggregate time as a group. It also helped to show us where we wanted to spend more time. Based on that, we worked together to better allocate our time. One of the things we decided to do was to each spend more time with patients, just shadowing them in their journey.

The way we accomplished this was by working with the site for which we had primary connection, and working with that site lead to identify a unit or an area where it would make sense to spend some extra time. We'd schedule a morning or an afternoon to be there, and then work with the staff to identify a patient who might be willing to allow us to be with him or her. We were a bit partial to finding patients without any family present so that our observation time could also serve the purpose of providing some friendly visiting to patients who may have otherwise been lonely. With patients' permission, we would then spend time with them in their day.

We would identify cool things as well as opportunities within the team interactions with the patients. We'd always be sure to debrief our time and experiences with the patient experience site lead. I'll never forget one example that proved very helpful to a site. This was in an inpatient med-surg unit, and my team member was paired up with a gentleman for the morning. Each time the staff entered the room, they would put their name on the care board and they'd say to the patient, "I'm going to put my name up here for you." My team member thought this was great, as there had been a big push to get staff to use the care boards in the rooms. After the third or fourth person had entered the room and done this, the patient leaned over to my team member and said, "I know they keep writing on something, but I'm not sure what it is. I'm legally blind so I can't read whatever they are writing on. Can you see it?"

This was terrific insight, and it led to discussions between my team member and the site lead about other patients who may not be able to see the care boards without their glasses, etc. Together they worked with the staff to reinforce the importance of not just writing a name on the care board, but introducing yourself to the patient. It may look something like this: "Hi, Mrs. Smith, I'm Janiece and I'm your nurse for this morning. I'm just going to write my name up here on your care board in case you forget it later. Don't worry, there's not a quiz, but we do have a whole team of people that you'll meet throughout today."

Authority and latitude

Regardless of whether you have a team or person and whether they are dedicated or designated with these roles, it is important to recognize what level of influence they can have across an organization. When I was working with my dream team for patient experience (the group of six that I've mentioned before), we talked a lot about how to influence without authority. We had accountability for the improvements in patient experience across the system, but we didn't have the authority over each individual to make that happen. As a department, we were a recognized resource and lead for this work in a large system. And we needed to get a big group of people to improve their local scores and care to make that happen. Our style was to partner and work collaboratively with the component parts of the system versus mandating "thou shalts" from the ivory tower.

Now, this does not mean that I'm not for standardization; we'll talk more about how to achieve that in later sections. However, I just want to acknowledge that the work in patient experience and patient- and family-centered care requires great skills in influencing and collaborating more so than just mandating and telling. Depending on how the positions are structured, the person or team leading patient experience can be situated in a dynamic where they have accountability for results without the complete authority to make that happen. As with many areas, the people who help determine our success are outside of our direct purview.

Chapter 6

Executive Sponsorship

One of the critical aspects to the success of the patient experience efforts in any organization is the senior leadership support for the work. I'm not just talking about the CEO—that person is obviously important. Depending on the size of the organization, it is usually a good idea to have someone else besides the CEO serving as the patient experience champion for the organization from a senior team perspective. Don't get me wrong: The CEO is an important champion of the patient experience efforts of the organization. However, I find that it's helpful to have more than just the CEO passionate about this work.

In organizations where there is a CXO, that person serves as the executive sponsor. In organizations without a CXO, another executive sponsor should be identified. The role of the executive sponsor is to provide support to the patient experience team and/or manager/director who are directly doing much of the work in the organization. Like any other initiative, the role of the patient experience executive sponsor is to help provide senior team visibility and support for the work. This person is also crucial to helping address barriers, bridge silos, and resolve interdepartmental issues.

While it may sound simple to name someone as the executive sponsor, finding the right person can be a rather difficult task that is sometimes underestimated in an organization. Over the years I've worked with many executive sponsors in various organizations. Based on that, I've come up with two key aspects that I think are most important to consider when identifying the right person to sponsor patient experience efforts in your organization:

1. Law of Motion

2. "It's more important who you are than what you do"

The Law of Motion

Newton's first law of motion is often stated as:

> *An object at rest stays at rest and an object in motion stays in motion with the same speed and in the same direction unless acted upon by an unbalanced force.* (The Physics Classroom, 2016)

I remember first learning about this principle in high school. The way this was explained to me was that it takes more energy to get a ball rolling than to redirect one that is already in motion.

While working with a series of four executive sponsors for patient experience in three years in one organization, I really recognized this principle. By the way, if that level of changing leadership doesn't give you whiplash, I don't know what will. Each one had their unique gifts and style and played a key role in the shaping of the work within the organization. As you might expect, each one took the agenda in a slightly different direction. As you can imagine, they each had different styles of leadership: A few leaned more toward the micromanaging, idea-a-minute type of activity, and one was more laid-back and hands off but still very active and wanting to lead it. Finally, it was the last one that really put me over the edge and helped me see this law of motion in action.

This fourth executive sponsor inherited patient experience right after a very high-energy, constant-ideas executive sponsor had just left the organization. The previous executive sponsor tended toward some micromanagement and almost a pace-setting type of style (constantly on to the next idea even before the last goal had been reached), and I thought that would be the most challenging personality and leader for me to work with on this. But I was wrong. The fourth executive sponsor was so unengaged, I felt like I'd slammed into a brick wall after going 75 miles per hour. I knew of this person in the organization and that the person was pretty likable, so I thought I could figure out

Chapter 6

how to work with the person and help keep the momentum that the previous executive sponsor had put into place. Once again, I was wrong.

This fourth executive sponsor embodied the principles of this law of motion. Over time, what I learned (in my frustration) was that it took more energy for me to try to get them to care about patient experience and to step up to try to lead it than it did for me to try to keep up with the previous sponsor's bundle of constant ideas and energy! I found myself yearning for that energy and enthusiasm. I realized that with that high-energy patient experience sponsor, I sometimes had to help redirect and shape the previous sponsor's ideas (at times it felt like a game of improv: "Yes … and"), but I later longed for that because of the amount of energy I had to incorporate to get the fourth sponsor to care and act.

"It's more important who you are than what you do"

One of my key mentors in high school was constantly helping to instill this into me. His point, at the time, was to help us figure out who we were as people and not be so defined by our activities (sports, music, theatre, etc.). I've thought of this often with the executive sponsors that I've seen in various organizations. The way I see this applied is in watching various leaders and where they are congruent with their hearts and actions. So many leaders can give lip service to the patient experience. Part of what I love about this field is that the case for caring is fun to talk about. However, true leadership and success in this area requires more than just lip service.

I've seen leaders do so much more harm than good in an organization by espousing the right terms/phrases and then ramrodding an agenda or being so forceful in their implementation of the tactics that they turn the organization off to the very work that they are trying to lead. Others are criticized for saying it's all about the patients, but then really focusing most of their time on the numbers of patient experience: the scores, etc.

To truly lead and champion this work, I think there has to be a congruency of words and actions, and to me that manifests itself in the person of the executive sponsor/leader. When this authentic congruency emerges, people see it, they are drawn to it, and they want to work and to help contribute to where this leader is headed. It's one thing for an executive sponsor who may be a physician to say to the docs, "We're going to use chairs to sit down when we talk to our patients." And it's another to fight to help get extra funding for stools or chairs and to lead by example and use them themselves!

This concept of congruency is true not just of the executive sponsors for this work but also for the patient experience leader and department who do the day-to-day work within the organization. I think one of the best summaries of what it takes to be a good leader comes from Colleen Sweeney in *The Hospital Leader Check List: 100 Characteristics of Top Leaders* (2014).

Leadership is about three things:

1. What you say, not what your name badge says.

2. What you do, not what you tell others to do.

3. Who you are … all day long.

It takes a village

I believe in the village principle of needing more people than just the CEO, the executive sponsor, and a patient experience leader to care about patient experience in an organization. To truly transform a culture, and make meaningful improvements in service and patient experience, it takes a village.

One of the best ways to create this village is to form some component of a steering committee to lead and carry out the patient experience efforts in the organization. I always advocate for the presence of one to three patients (who also serve on one of the Patient and Family Advisory Councils), several frontline staff, and leaders from around the organization led by a dyad of the executive sponsor and the leader for patient experience. Again, I like to apply those principles of congruency and inertia/motion to finding people to serve on this committee. Finding those who truly have a genuine passion for the work is important and can help to really make these efforts blossom throughout the organization.

Regardless of care setting (hospital, clinic, ED, surgery center, long-term care, home health, or hospice), I find it helpful to identify some subcommittees focused on key aspects related to that group's core purpose. For example, if pain management and communication with nurses are two key composites for a hospital, I'd suggest having subgroups focused on that. Or, if access and communication with doctors are two important aspects for a clinic, have subgroups focused on those efforts. It may be the environmental services director leading this as a subcommittee in a long-term care facility or organization where environmental cleanliness is a noted area of opportunity.

In these situations, I look for a steering team member who has a particular interest and natural affinity for that work to partner with the patient experience leader or other team member to lead that group. These subcommittees usually meet outside or in addition to the steering team meetings to get some of their group's work done. They then report out to the larger steering team at their meetings.

What to Look For in a Patient Experience Leader

Patient experience is not about *a* person or *a* team. If that's how the organization is looking at this work, it will not succeed. Patient experience is a movement, and it is a culture that needs to flow throughout the organization. While it's not about the person or the people who you choose to lead this for your organization, I would be remiss if I didn't highlight how important it is to select the right person or the right people for those roles.

Assuming you've secured some level of resources to dedicate or even designate someone to lead patient experience for your organization, what are you looking for in that person? It's not an easy task—although it is getting easier. Thanks to the work of places like the Beryl Institute and the Institute for Patient- and Family-Centered Care, there has been a movement created and a profession is really emerging. I was pleased to be part of the first cohort of Certified Patient Experience Professionals (CPXP) by the Patient Experience Institute in 2016. Regardless of certification, finding people who want to do this work is easier now than it has been ever before.

In the past two years, I have attended large patient experience symposiums with two of my team members, who both hail from the IT side of healthcare. As part of our work together, they've been branching out from the data component of patient experience and working in areas of coaching, training, and improvement. As part of that, I'd asked them each to attend a patient experience conference. After this, I'd thanked them for attending, acknowledging that it was outside of their typical focus and training/natural comfort zone. They both remarked on how there was such a personality about the people they encountered at these conferences. They found it very easy to sit down in a session and just strike up a conversation with someone about patient experience and their work. They said, "Janiece, these people are so fun! This is *not* like the IT conferences that we go to!"

The people who are drawn to this patient experience field come from many different places. The ideal person who you want to lead this work across an organization does need to have an engaging personality and a passion for the work that they do. This doesn't mean that they have to be overly charismatic or inspiring, although that's a plus; it just means that they need to be able to connect with others with some enthusiasm that engages others in the work.

Chapter 6

When I first started in consulting, I was talking to a dear friend about feeling slightly intimidated about sales. I told her, "All I ever sold were Girl Scout cookies!" My friend had been in consulting for quite a while and had recently joined a startup; her advice was so true. She said, "Don't think of it as sales; think of it as just talking with people about what you're passionate about. When you tell them the stories of the work that you do, your natural energy and enthusiasm for that will come out and they'll be drawn to it." I've learned that she was absolutely right. This same thing is true for those who are leading patient experience efforts; they need not be "selling" patient experience to the frontline staff, leaders, and physicians in the organization, but they do need to be able to articulate with some level of energy and enthusiasm about the difference this work can make for the patients and families they serve.

When I am asked to help an organization create a position or hire someone to lead patient experience in their organizations, we work through the somewhat obvious aspects that you may expect:

- Ability to speak in front of others

- Ability to write and tell stories

- Ability to relate to patients and families, frontline staff, leaders, physicians

I also help them to define and look for many of the intangibles that may not always lend themselves to job description aspects. Many of these need to surface in interview questions and in talking to references and colleagues who have worked with this person before. Let's take a look at a few of them.

Desire to defy the asymptote

Asymp … what? Yep, I'm going to take you back to high school math. An *asymptote* is a mathematical term for an imaginary line (or a limit) that an equation approaches but never quite touches. Consider the graph in Figure

Setting Up for Success

6.3. On the left side of the graph, no matter how big X gets, Y will get closer and closer to the asymptote but never reach it. Call me a geek, but I and many of the people that I work with use this as a concept as a tongue-in-cheek way to describe healthcare challenges that seem impossible to overcome. Together with some fellow geeks, we liked this concept so much that we used it in the name of our consulting company, DTA Associates, Inc. (i.e., Defy the Asymptote).

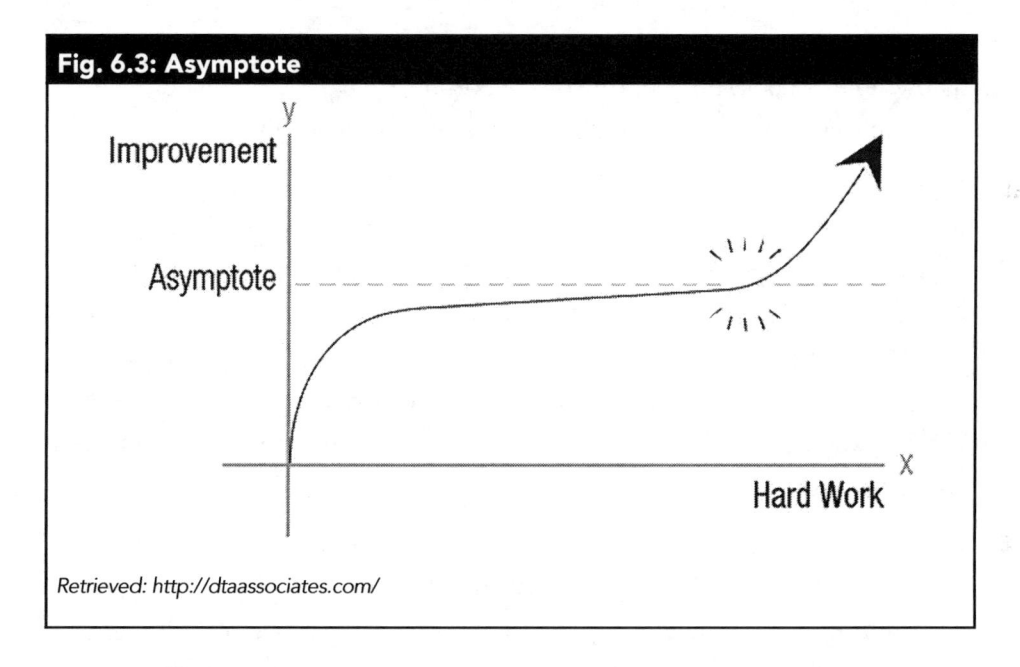

Fig. 6.3: Asymptote

Retrieved: http://dtaassociates.com/

For many organizations, their asymptote may be their patient experience scores that have plateaued. Or the litany of projects that go on forever never seem to attain the intended results and instead frustrate teams. Whatever it is, the only way to overcome an asymptote is to defy it (like on the right side of the graph), just like you would defy gravity.

What in the world does this have to do with what to look for in a patient experience leader? Well, you're looking for people who have the desire to defy an asymptote. Making vast improvements in patient experience or changing the culture of an organization to be more service-oriented are not easy things to accomplish. They are not for the faint of heart, and they take a lot of perseverance. It can feel like defying gravity, and it takes someone who truly desires to do it to make that happen!

Desire (or not) for structure

I am a planner—I love to see where I'm going. I like to map things out months and sometimes years in advance. I'm a list maker and a project planner. Even as I write this book, I'm working off an outline; I have a deadline for when the manuscript is due. Within there I have set page goals for myself each time I sit down to write. Type A? Yep, you guessed it!

Furthermore, I was trained in Lean and I have a black belt in Six Sigma. Not only can I project manage with the best of them but I can also get into the weeds on statistics if I have to. Many people who come out of a similar background as me struggle with working in patient experience. I've seen plenty of people with my credentials (minus the social work) struggle to succeed in patient experience unless they can set aside some of their need for detail and traditional process improvement where $x + y = z$.

Don't get me wrong, I don't think that all process improvement in healthcare is by any means linear, easy, or straightforward. That being said, process improvement in patient experience requires taking a bit of a different approach. Where I have found success and when I have seen others have it is when they can take the best parts of what they know from Lean, PDSA, Six Sigma, etc., and bring all of that in their toolbox and pull out the elements that fit, when required.

When looking for a leader for patient experience work, often we look to the ranks of quality and performance improvement. To be fair, when I led a whole department of patient experience program managers, we had the requirement that they each had at least a green belt in Six Sigma. We wanted that knowledge and understanding of performance improvement. This becomes important when working with improvement efforts and balancing communication and efficiency. For example, I'm able to assure the physicians and staff that I work with that I'm an efficiency expert. It pains me to ever suggest anything that will take them more time in the long run. When I ask them to alter their communication style, I do so sharing how it will help to improve their efficiency over time.

The shadow side to these skills can be the desire for structure, clarity, and more detail than sometimes is available in the patient experience world. It's possible to make that transition as I have, but I've also seen some people really struggle to make that jump. When someone who desires more of a typical performance improvement project finds their way into patient experience, they can be frustrated, and that can lead to less than desirable results. If you're interviewing someone coming from this background, ask them to describe the differences between patient experience improvement and traditional performance improvement in healthcare. This will help you to look at whether or not he or she has thought about this and allow you to probe further about how the person sees him- or herself making that transition.

Ability to handle ambiguity

Regardless of the background and training of the person you hire to lead patient experience in your organization, it is essential that they be able to handle ambiguity. There's no silver bullet to magically improve the patient experience. There are some essential steps, which we will cover in future chapters, but there is no easy fix. The reality is that organizations that have succeeded in this space have devoted significant amounts of time and resources and have had to try some things (plural) to achieve their success.

It is essential that you are looking for a person who is willing to go the distance and be in this with your organization for the long haul. Understanding the person's vision, sense of timing for improvement, and asking him or her about what one thing could make the most difference for the organization is

Chapter 6

patient experience are helpful ways to understand where this person is at on this aspect.

Gentle but firm

Another criterion to look for in a patient experience leader is someone who is gentle, approachable, kind—the face of patient experience, but who is also able to be firm. Going in front of groups of physicians who are angry about CMS and value-based purchasing is not for a meek and mild person. It is super-important to hear them out and also gently find a way to still toe the line of necessary improvement. Ideally, the patient experience leader will also be able to infuse humor at the appropriate moments and won't shy away from a hearty discussion of concerns by care team members.

Success = Working yourself out of a job

An essential characteristic of a patient experience leader is a humble acknowledgment that one of the best things that could happen would be to work him- or herself out of a job. When I led my dream team for patient experience, we all acknowledged that the best thing that would happen would be that the organization would hit all of its goals and that the culture would change such that we would no longer be needed in our roles! Over time, that's exactly what happened. That same thing is true for me today in the consulting world. It may sound weird for someone running a consulting firm to say, but part of how we define success is when the organization we've consulted with is in a place to succeed without us. If we step away and all of the work falls apart, then we haven't truly done our jobs.

People who truly "get" patient experience understand that there could be no greater honor than to no longer be needed in an organization because the work is moving ahead at the staff, unit, and local levels. A great way to see where a potential candidate is at on this is to ask how he or she would define success in this role.

Relationship with data

Patient experience is not all about the data—but you can't be successful in this work without being savvy about data. When interviewing people for roles in patient experience, I like to ask them a bit about their relationship with data: Are they data geeks? Do they see it as a necessary evil? Do they rely on analysts for most of it? Where are they on this spectrum?

When I first got involved with patient experience, I was coming out of the performance improvement arm of an organization and had gotten my black belt, etc. But if I'm honest, it took me a while to get my head around some of the aspects of the patient experience data. Tracy Laibson painstakingly and patiently walked me through the difference between percentage top box and percentile again and again.

The data is an important part of this work; it's not the most important part, but a knowledge and command of it is essential. We're going to spend some time working through the issues and challenges as well as some of the ways to use and succeed with the data in the coming chapters.

I never was more convinced of the importance of a patient experience leader's approach to the data than when I was working with a new patient experience director. This person was used to more timely metrics in some of the Lean projects that work that the director had previously led. The person looked to the patient experience data available to use in the same manner, and became frustrated. I'll never forget the day that this person looked at me and exclaimed, "I hate HCAHPS data!" Frustration with CMS and the lag in the data from improvements, these issues I understand—but you can't fundamentally hate the data that helps to define your success. Needless to say, this person wasn't in that role for much longer, realizing that this frustration was also affecting others in the process.

Bottom line: You need someone who has a healthy relationship with the data to lead this work. Lack of confidence or frustration with the data will not help in engaging physicians and other leaders in this area.

As you can see with all of these aspects at play, there are many things to look for in finding the right leader to shepherd the patient experience efforts within your organization.

References

Barnet, S. (2015). 7 things to know about CXO salaries. Retrieved June 27, 2016, from *www.beckershospitalreview.com/compensation-issues/7-things-to-know-about-cxo-salaries.html*

Padilla, D. (2014). The Chief Experience Officer. Retrieved June 27, 2016, from *http://healthcare-executive-insight.advanceweb.com/Features/Articles/The-Chief-Experience-Officer.aspx*

Sweeney, C. (2014). *The Hospital Leader Check List – 100 Characteristics of Top Leaders.* Sweeney Healthcare Enterprises.

The Physics Classroom. (2016). Newton's laws—Lesson 1—Newton's first law of motion. Retrieved June 27, 2016, from *www.physicsclassroom.com/class/newtlaws/Lesson-1/Newton-s-First-Law*

Wolf, J. A., and Prince, D. (2014). *The Chief Experience Officer—An Emerging & Critical Role.* The Beryl Institute.

Section 4
Data

As we discussed in the last chapter, data is a key component to success in improving patient- and family-centered care. While it is not the most important aspect, it's a significant one, with many facets that are critical to your organization's achievement of your goals. Data factors heavily into the compulsories, it is a key way in which we can connect with physicians in particular, and it is obviously essential to measuring the efforts employed in collaboration. In this section we are going to talk about various sources, challenges, and important ways to use data to help hold the organization accountable to key goals in the patient experience space.

Chapter 7
Sources of Data and Supporting Technology

by Kevin Campbell and Janiece Gray

One of the first things to consider with regard to data is the various sources of patient experience data within the organization. In previous sections we've talked about various aspects of the patients' voices to project, and one of the best places where these patient comments can be found is the open-ended questions on any survey.

In addition to comments, there is plenty of quantitative data related to the patient experience. Most organizations, regardless of sector (long-term care, home health, emergency department, ambulatory surgery centers, clinics, hospitals) have some kind of survey related to their patients' experiences. In many cases, there are requirements about this: HCAHPS, CG CAHPS, HH CAHPS, and ICH CAHPS. One of the biggest considerations for organizations is whether to survey the minimum required both in terms of sample size and frequency. For meaningful improvement, it's often necessary to go beyond these minimum requirements or to augment these required tools with other tools and technology. In other organizations, even those without a requirement for a survey, most have determined the need for some component of measurement on the pulse of their patients and families or residents' experiences. Many organizations that were early adopters in using the tools before they became required often are far ahead in terms of performance when reporting becomes a mandate.

Types of Measures

There are three types of outcomes used to help judge success on a project (Institute of Healthcare Improvement, n.d.). These measures are:

1. Outcome

2. Balancing

3. Process

The outcome measure is really your target for improvement. For example, in patient experience, the survey results that are publicly reported are used to calculate value-based purchasing as the outcome measure.

The balancing measure is the metric that you look at to make sure that improvement in one area doesn't negatively impact another. If we are asking nurses to do a bedside shift report, we don't want to negatively impact overtime. In this case, overtime would be the balancing measure.

The process measure is specific to the processes or strategies that lead to success in the overall outcome. If the communication composite is the outcome, some process measures may include specific strategies around use of care boards in the rooms or rounding on patients.

Most often, the survey data or outcome measure is what is focused on in the organization. We will spend some significant time talking about that and the challenges and successes in using those data. Later, we will also look at some options for tracking and trending process measures while being mindful of balancing measures.

Survey Partner

Our first exposure to patient experience was in working with an organization where the organization was its own vendor for its required surveys. This involved following the specifications from CMS related to sending surveys, opening the mail, date stamping, and scanning in the surveys within a certain time frame. It also involved numerous quality checks of the equipment, etc. As we worked through the need for improvement in the organization, we determined that 90% of our time was being spent identifying the patients, sending the surveys, getting the surveys, scanning the surveys, and reporting the surveys, and only 5%–10% of our time was left for understanding the data that we had and making steps toward meaningful improvement.

Consequently, we decided to outsource our survey administration to a partner. We incorporated a patient in the request for proposal (RFP) process and he, together with an interdisciplinary team of leaders, helped us to select a survey partner. This process occurred very quickly within a six-week implementation timeline.

For the required surveys, there are a ton of quality checks and various other requirements that are arduous for an organization to manage themselves. We definitely advocate for outsourcing this function. However, simply turning this over to a survey vendor does not eliminate the need for leaders within the organization to know what is going on with the data.

When we led the RFP process to outsource the surveying, we carefully chose the language of "survey partner." Moving away from the use of the term "vendor." It sounds like semantics, but it's really deliberate language aimed at creating a partnership that is essential to success and improvement in this arena. If you don't have a partnership with your survey company, then you need to intentionally forge one. The reason this is so essential is that you and the teams that you work with (the physicians in particular) need to trust the data.

Chapter 7

We'll talk about some of the challenges inherent to patient experience data in general, but you need not add any concerns regarding data quality to those.

The Grass is Always Greener

In our work today at DTA, we are often asked to come in and help organizations lead their own RFP process as they look to switch companies or explore switching companies for their surveys. For this reason, we try to stay neutral with regard to any endorsement of one vendor over another. What we can tell you is this: In countless organizations that we work with on improvement, we will hear complaints about their survey vendor. The reality is that at this point, we've heard complaints about pretty much every company out there. These complaints generally center on certain themes:

- Data quality
- Frequent turnover of account reps assigned to the organization
- Lack of timely responses to questions or concerns
- Feeling like you're a big fish in a small pond or feeling like you're a small fish in a big pond (this is mostly in regard to benchmarks and time and attention from the survey company)
- Survey mode adjustments (transition from mail to email, or to phone or Interactive Voice Response, etc.)

The fact that we've heard these complaints about pretty much every survey company out there leads us to counsel organizations that when they are looking to make a switch to remember that the grass is always greener on the other vendor's side of the fence. There is a cost to switching vendors—mostly on the backs of your report writers, data warehouse team, and data analysts—but also in terms of retraining the organization on how data is displayed, how reports can be retrieved, etc. That being said, sometimes that's the only way to start fresh and realize the goal of forming a new survey partnership.

Supplement to Aid in Improvement

Regardless of your vendor partner, we encourage organizations to take advantage of their proprietary survey items. On the required surveys (HCAHPS, CG CAHPS, HH CAHPS, etc.), organizations have the option to add some key items to the survey. This makes many people uncomfortable about the length of the survey. We hear that and will still encourage that you consider even up to 10 supplemental items that can help to inform your improvement. For example, if you're focused on communication—items about courtesy and respect, listening carefully, and explaining things really only tell you so much. There are much more comprehensive items that can drill down into more specifics that help you know where to focus with your care team (see Figure 7.1).

Consider this example for the Communication with Doctors composite within HCAHPS. We love this because it really helps to inform the greater areas of detail within communication. Most every vendor has their own proprietary survey items to add in addition to your CAHPS-required surveys. By going beyond the compulsories, you're able to start to connect the dots to really lead to collaborative improvement. The other thing that this can do is to help identify and track some of the hidden composites that can help impact CAHPS performance. Look at how the teamwork and coordination of information between the care team is so essential to the patients' perceptions of their physicians' communication.

Chapter 7

Fig. 7.1: Proprietary Survey

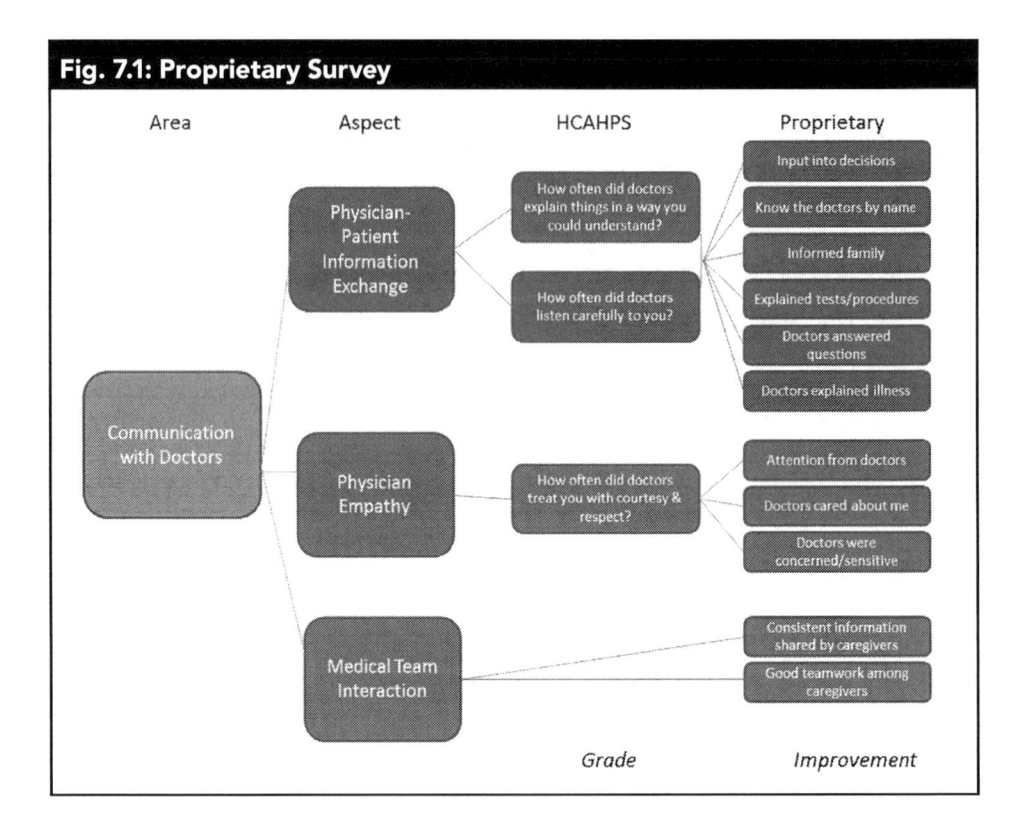

Area	Aspect	HCAHPS	Proprietary
Communication with Doctors	Physician-Patient Information Exchange	How often did doctors explain things in a way you could understand? How often did doctors listen carefully to you?	Input into decisions Know the doctors by name Informed family Explained tests/procedures Doctors answered questions Doctors explained illness
	Physician Empathy	How often did doctors treat you with courtesy & respect?	Attention from doctors Doctors cared about me Doctors were concerned/sensitive
	Medical Team Interaction		Consistent information shared by caregivers Good teamwork among caregivers
		Grade	Improvement

Augment With Appropriate Technology to Inform

Regardless of the survey tool that you use to meet the current or coming requirements for your service area/organization, it is often very helpful to augment these with additional sources of data. While the survey tool that you use to report to whatever public agency you need to may comprise your outcome metrics, there are many other ways to get process metrics for the organization. Another reason that organizations will use additional sources of technology to inform their work is due to the timing of the responses. The key here is to be careful that questions asked while a patient is still an inpatient, for example, do not resemble the questions on the HCAHPS survey.

Specifically, "HCAHPS should be the first survey patients receive about their experience of hospital care." CMS is very serious that organizations adhere to this (2009).

That being said, there are still ways you can get more real-time feedback from patients. A great way to do this is to spot-check an improvement. Let's say that you implemented a new care board in the emergency department and you want to know how it's being used and how patients perceive it. Finding a way to ask questions about that on a quick kiosk or in-room tablet technology for a few weeks or months can help you to see how your improvement is progressing.

We like to stay neutral with regard to these technology companies as much as with the survey companies. In this space, there are more and more companies with varying technology popping up all the time. There are some excellent products out there that we have used in various organizations, so you have many good options to consider.

Rounding Tools

Another key place where technology can help to augment your efforts is with regard to rounding. Whether you're rounding in an inpatient unit, a long-term care facility, or the waiting room of an emergency department or clinic, there are plenty of applications of rounding both on staff and on patients. We would never say that you have to have an electronic tool or tablet to make this happen—simple pen and paper will do. However, to really make it efficient for the supervisors, managers, and even the volunteers who you may train to do this in the organization, having some sort of assistive technology can be crucial to the tracking, trending, and long-term adoption of this practice.

Part of the reason we do advocate for some kind of application that tracks information on rounding is because of a particularly poignant experience

Chapter 7

we had in one organization. This hospital system was rolling out rounding for their leaders on patients; however, they did not yet have a tracking tool. Janiece was doing some coaching with the leaders who were doing the rounding to help them maximize the effectiveness of their time spent rounding. In the morning, she was shadowing the med-surg manager and had a delightful conversation with one woman, Ahna (not her real name). Later that afternoon, she was shadowing and coaching with the director of environmental services (EVS), who was also supposed to be rounding on patients on various units. Before she knew it and could stop it, they were back in Ahna's room! Ahna was just delightful and they had such a great conversation, they ended up recruiting this patient to be part of the Patient and Family Advisory Group.

Not everyone is as kind as Ahna. If there is no way for the director of EVS to know that the manager of the unit was in there just that morning, everyone looks like they're tripping over each other. Plus, it gets frustrating to the patients to be answering the same questions and having time taken away from their rest and healing. And what if Ahna had raised a concern with the manager that morning? When the EVS director walked in that afternoon, she'd have no idea about it and Ahna would have to tell her about it again—it would look like the manager was not listening earlier in the day. In focus groups with patients, they talk about how exhausting it is to have to tell their story over and over.

After this, whenever rounding on patients in an organization without any tracking tools, we first find the manager and ask about any patients to be sure to visit or not to visit. If the manager is doing the rounding, we also encourage them to check in with the nurse before walking into the room. There may be various reasons to not round on a patient on a given day. On one oncology unit, the manager said that the patient had just had a really tough night, had been awake a lot, and was finally getting some much needed rest.

The organization where Janiece first met Ahna eventually adopted an electronic tool for tracking their rounding. This greatly aided them in not only addressing the redundancies and making sure they knew if that patient had already been rounded on or not but it also allowed them to track and trend how many of their patients they were able to round on. As they had key aspects that they were focused on (e.g., food service, care boards, new bedside practices), they were able to prompt questions for those doing the rounding to gather feedback from the patients and families about these aspects. They were also able to easily notify other departments if there was a service alert or to work together to help make something special happen for the patients and families, which is exactly what happened one Wednesday to Janiece.

> *On that Wednesday, I was rounding on the oncology unit where the manager had identified a few patients who would be good for me to visit. I went to the first room and met this nice gentleman and his wife. He was scheduled to have surgery that day, but they agreed to speak with me for a few moments. They spoke so highly of the care that they had received, saying things like, "I can't remember who they all are, but one woman stands out in particular who took care of me several days in a row," or "The people who bring the food, the people who clean the room. The staff, everyone has been great about introducing themselves and telling us their role and what they are there to do."*
>
> *In the course of our short conversation, they shared a bit about this last year's journey and how rough it had been for them. The surgery the patient was having was pretty major but they were excited to finally have it. They had been working for months at various other hospitals, trying to figure out what was wrong. Somewhere during all of that he had been in the hospital for an entire month. They were so pleased to be at this facility and to finally have some answers and a course of treatment.*
>
> *As I was saying goodbye, I thanked them for the chance to talk with them and for their feedback. I made a comment that I enjoyed meeting them and just wished it wouldn't have had to be in the hospital.*

Chapter 7

They agreed and quipped something about the fact that their 27th anniversary was Friday, and they would still be here for that. I connected with that, in part because their anniversary is exactly one week before mine!

I was tracking their feedback in the new rounding tool and saw a way to make a note to food service. I decided to just see if and how it would work and made a note about Friday being their 27th anniversary and how cool it would be to surprise them with something special. Well, it worked! The note ultimately made it to the director of food service, who, along with her team, worked some magic.

I also made sure to let the manager know just because I thought she would want to know in case she could acknowledge it on Friday. After that, I flew back to Minnesota and didn't think much more of it. That Friday, I received an email from the manager that said: Picture of the anniversary party on a cart! Thank you for putting this on your rounding form. The patient and wife were truly touched!

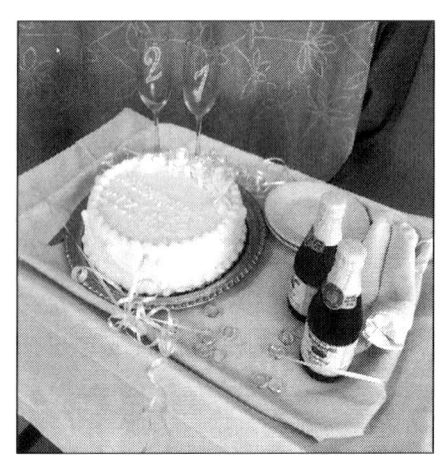

When I saw the photo of what had happened, it brought tears to my eyes. I never imagined such a beautiful display honoring this special day for this wonderful couple. Did you see the glasses? They have a 2 and a 7 on them for their 27th anniversary. The food service director and her team are to be commended for an excellent job.

> *It made me so proud to be associated with such an amazing group of people who were willing to exceed their patients' expectations, especially in such difficult circumstances.*
>
> *Now, did they have to have a rounding tool to make this happen? Absolutely not! I could have made a note to remember to email the food service director and to tell the manager and it all could have still happened. However, think of the countless missed opportunities to do things like this just because we forget or don't take the time to remember to send an email. The more automated we can make the systems and tools to help us achieve on the patient experience we wish to deliver, the better.*

The Electronic Medical Record

When you think about supportive technologies related to patient experience, your electronic medical record (EMR) system probably doesn't immediately jump to mind. It's kind of like the electrical wiring in your house: what it delivers is essential to your guests enjoying themselves at your dinner party, but it only gets noticed if it stops doing what it's supposed to do. And it's okay if your patients don't notice your EMR exists. That means it is doing its job. But you shouldn't fail to take your EMR into consideration as you seek to improve the experience of your patients.

There are various ways your EMR can directly affect the patient experience:

- Reducing the amount of time patients have to wait. For instance, effective use of order sets can allow a patient's labs and consultations to be ordered quicker and therefore get completed quicker.

- Facilitating patient comfort. Optimizing alerts and alarms can allow patients to relax more—nurses aren't the only ones who get alarm fatigue!

Chapter 7

- Improving communication. When clinicians are able to document quickly, and their coworkers are able to find that documentation easily, key messages get to where they need to go to facilitate smooth transitions and proper care coordination. Patients expect their caregivers to all be reading off the same song sheet, and appreciate when it is being done well.

- Finally, when designed, supported, and explained to your patients properly, increasing the convenience of interacting with your organization. An automated appointment reminder that helps mom and dad remember their child's school vaccination appointment goes a long way in helping out an already busy schedule. Your more tech-savvy patients are going to appreciate an easy-to-use patient portal that allows them to view lab results and make appointments without having to pick up a phone.

In this chapter, we've covered quite a few sources of data to consider incorporating in your improvement efforts. We initially looked at many of the types of measures to be mindful of when making improvements. We looked at several sources outside of the standard survey data including technology for real-time feedback and rounding tools as well as the electronic medical record. The survey partner that your organization selects is very important to the quality and availability of data that you have—not only for the standardized/required surveys but also for the additional items that you can add to aid in improvement. In the next section, we'll take a look at the ways in which you can display and act upon your organization's data.

References

Centers for Medicare & Medicaid Services. (2009). Retrieved June 27, 2016, from *www.hcahpsonline.org/files/2009-01%20HCAHPS%20Bulletin%202009-01%20Revised%205-15-2009.pdf*

Institute of Healthcare Improvement. (n.d.). Science of improvement: Establishing measures. Retrieved June 27, 2016, from *www.ihi.org/resources/Pages/HowtoImprove/ScienceofImprovementEstablishingMeasures.aspx*

Chapter 8
The Display and Use of Data

by Kevin Campbell

It can often seem like the work of patient experience is all about the data. You more than likely have encountered some of the following questions:

- "When will the data be available?"
- "How can I get to my department's data?"
- "Is this data accurate?"
- "How do we compare to like organizations?"
- "Are any of these organizations even like us at all?"
- "Did we hit our incentive goal last quarter?"
- "Did the right patients get attributed to me?"

With all that data, we can lose sight of the object of the data: the patient. This happens for various reasons, but here are a few:

- Lack of trust in the data—enough wrong data has made its way to meetings and companywide dashboards that the data has to be scrutinized

Chapter 8

- Nerd alert—healthcare is a scientific endeavor, and scientists like numbers, so the slicing and dicing of data can really flourish in such a habitat as healthcare

- "Rank and spank"*—When data is used as a stick to punish and/or embarrass people into doing better, they are going to end up paying excessive attention to the data (*hat tip to Dr. Jeff Vespa)

All of that being said, data is still very important in the patient experience world. Anecdotal evidence alone seems particularly inaccurate when it comes to our perceptions of how patients feel about our organization and the care we provide. So data is essential to help us see more clearly where we need to improve and even specifically how we need to improve.

In this chapter, we'll cover *some* best practices for the display and use of data with the intent of making data meaningful, helpful, and something upon which action is actually taken.

The first thing that needs to be addressed regarding the use of patient experience data is how leaders, providers, and analysts are going to access it. Your survey vendor (I mean partner) will certainly have reporting capabilities, and this is a good place to start. We live in an age where good-looking, easy-to-use, web-based self-service portals are no longer a premium add-on, but rather a basic expectation. And since survey data is relatively simple data to work with, as soon as surveys start coming in, your survey partner should be able to flip a switch and make some solid reports available to you. In addition, if your survey partner has a large client base, they will have at least some comparison data (percentiles) that can help prove that, yes, we do actually have areas in which we are not the best in the nation.

There are, however, some things to consider before rolling out your survey partner's website to everyone in the organization:

The Display and Use of Data

- Limited or no integration with other key data. Your survey partner will likely allow extra information to be submitted to them along with the basic data needed to generate and send a survey, but it will always mean additional work and waiting to get additional clinical and financial data displayed along with your patient experience data. If you bring your survey results into your own repository, you have many more options to marry that data with key organizational data.

- Yet another login to another website. It may not be the straw that breaks the camel's back, but the login information may get lost in the pile and be seen as more hassle than it's worth to your leaders.

- Nonstandard reporting functionality. Not only is it a hassle to have to maintain login information to yet another website, but it can also be inefficient and confusing for users to have to learn multiple visualization and reporting tools. If your organization is attempting to standardize reporting and visualization tools for efficiency and ease of training, your survey partner's offerings won't likely align well with those efforts.

So there are pros and cons of utilizing your survey partner's reports versus importing data into a local repository and using your own tools. Chances are that you will end up pursuing a combination of both approaches. You may choose to direct your leaders to your survey partner's website for survey results (especially percentiles) by nursing unit, but there will always be a need for patient experience scores to be displayed alongside your quality, operational, and financial performance on internal dashboards or scorecards. How much emphasis you put on either approach will vary depending on your internal capabilities to integrate and display data and your survey partner's capabilities to do the same.

Chapter 8

Percentiles

As I mentioned above, the desire for percentile data is a good reason to utilize your survey partner's website. Why is that? What is special about a vendor that they can offer percentiles and I can't do it internally? To answer that, let's spend a little time understanding the difference between percentiles and top-box scores, beginning with a definition of "top-box."

In CAHPS parlance, top-box scores are a measure of survey respondents giving the highest marks on a particular question. On a 4-point scale (Never/Sometimes/Usually/Always), "Always" or 4 is a top-box response. On a question with a 10-point scale, a response of 9 or 10 is considered top-box. Let's look at an example using the question "During this hospital stay, how often was the area around your room quiet at night?" which is a 4-point Never/Sometimes/Usually/Always question. Here are the results of that question for the 10 surveys returned:

Survey 1: Always (4)   Survey 6: Always (4)
Survey 2: Sometimes (2)   Survey 7: Usually (3)
Survey 3: Always (4)   Survey 8: Always (4)
Survey 4: Usually (3)   Survey 9: Sometimes (2)
Survey 5: Always (4)   Survey 10: Always (4)

The average response for the "quiet at night" question is:
(4 + 2 + 4 + 3 + 4 + 4 + 3 + 4 + 2 + 4)/10 = 3.4

An average of 3.4 is well above an overall "Usually" response. It doesn't seem like there is a lot of room for improvement there. However, the top-box score can be quite a bit more harsh. For questions on a 4-point scale, only responses of 4 count as top-box. In this example with six responses of "Always," the top box score is 6/10 or 60%. That's barely above half! Not nearly as encouraging as the average, but top-box scores are what are most often used, and therefore they are what we need to pay attention to. On the positive side, the bottom-box score (yes, that is a thing) is 0% since there were no responses of 1 (Never) given in this example.

Is 60% top-box good or bad? An average of 3.4 out of 4 seems good, but in school 60% is barely passing. It is difficult to know what constitutes "good" in a vacuum, so we look to others for comparisons, and that's where percentiles come in.

A percentile is an indication of where your survey population sits in comparison to a much larger population of surveys. In the case of the "quiet at night" example, a 60% top-box performance would put your organization a little below the 50th percentile of the 4,182 hospitals publicly reported by CMS for patients discharged between July 2014 and June 2015 (2016). The 50th percentile, which is equivalent to the median top-box score, was 62% top-box, which means half of the hospitals scored 62% or better, and half scored 62% or worse. So now you know that you are near the middle of the pack for how patients rate your hospital's quietness at night. However, it's worth noting that the 25th percentile is a 55% top-box score, so lose a few points and suddenly you are worse than 75% of hospitals.

Better Comparisons

Now, as your leaders, especially those in departments that can be either loud or quiet at night, look at the report that says the hospital is slightly worse than half the hospitals in the United States at being quiet, the objection that will undoubtedly arise is "We're being compared to hospitals that are totally different than ours." And they might be right. Maybe compared to similar-sized hospitals, they are performing very well.

CMS doesn't publish percentiles based on the size or type of hospital or other care setting. You can't compare yourself to large academic hospitals or small critical access hospitals. They also don't publish percentiles for every possible

Chapter 8

slice and dice of the data you might want to do—for instance, if you wanted to find out what percentile your med-surg unit falls into or how your primary care physicians rank against other primary care physicians. This is where your survey partner comes in.

Because your survey partner has multiple clients, their database of patient experience survey responses can help you see how you are doing compared to those other clients. However, not all survey vendors are the same in this regard. The larger and more geographically diverse the partner's client base, the more the benchmarks will reflect national performance. And the higher number of surveys in the database, the finer your comparisons can be (meaning hospital type or even specialty comparisons may be available). If you are working with a smaller or more regionalized partner, be aware that your percentile rankings are going to be less representative of your national standing. That isn't necessarily a bad thing, especially if you are in a high-performing region of the country and you want to be pushed to perform by the best of the best. The bottom line is to be aware of the data and comparisons available from by your survey partner.

Let's say you are working with a large survey partner with hundreds of clients scattered across the country. When you have a database of that size and good reporting and visualization functionality, it's possible to calculate percentiles at all sorts of levels of analysis. You may be asked, "How do we compare on specific DRGs or amongst various age groups or races?" However, just because you *can* get percentiles at every dimension doesn't mean you *should* pay attention to them all. The further you drill into your data, the fewer comparative survey responses there will be, even with a large population. For example, if you drill down to an obscure DRG, how many of your survey partner's clients provide that service, and what volume of survey responses fall into that DRG? If you are being percentile-ranked on 10 surveys in addition to your own, that isn't overly helpful. So keep an eye on the sample size.

The Display and Use of Data

Another issue with excessive focus on percentile rankings at every level of data analysis is it can distract from improvement. **If our response to unfavorable percentile rankings is to continually ask for finer and finer comparisons, there's a good chance we're trying to avoid having to be accountable to making changes to increase patient satisfaction in those areas.** The best way to use percentiles is to look at them when setting goals, and then move forward in improvement with a focus on the goals. Percentiles help us set reasonable goals, but from there we should keep our focus on improving from wherever we are at. This also helps us avoid drilling down further and further until we find a number we "can live with."

The final problem we'll discuss related to utilizing percentiles is that insistence on viewing percentile data on internal reports can cause a significant challenge. We have seen this issue play out at multiple organizations where survey data is downloaded from the survey partner to be displayed using the organization's internal reporting and visualization tools. Percentiles are easy to calculate when you have the full survey response population at your disposal (like your survey partner does). It is simply lining up the average scores for each organization for a particular survey question, and then calculating the percentile cutoffs (25th percentile = 25% of organizations score at or below that amount).

However, when you are working with only your own organization's data, you can no longer calculate percentiles. The best you can do is map percentile data that's been given to you. Recall our earlier example for the "quiet at night" HCAHPS survey question: We calculated a 60% top-box score. Then we compared that to a table of percentiles published by CMS and found that 60% put us between the 25th percentile (55%) and the 50th percentile (62%). One of the limitations of this approach is that it lacks specificity (we don't have incremental percentiles between 25 and 50). This can be dealt with in a couple of ways, one of which is interpolating the percentiles to approximate our exact percentile. Here's how that's done:

Chapter 8

50th percentile – 25th percentile = 25 percentiles
62% top-box (50th percentile) – 55% top-box (25th percentile) = 7% top-box difference
25 percentiles / 7% = 3.57 percentiles per 1% top-box
60% (our score) – 55% (25th percentile) = 5% above the 25th
5 * 3.57 = 17.85 steps above the 25th percentile

17.85 + 25 = 42.85
42.85 rounded to the nearest integer = the **43rd percentile**

The main mathematical problem with this approach is that percentiles for patient experience data will never be linear—in fact, they are more likely to conform more closely to a bell-shaped curve—and the above method assumes linearity. So if your organization is paying close attention to every percentile gain (or loss), interpolating the actual percentile between two percentiles may not be telling an accurate story.

The preferable approach if you are focusing in on the slightest percentile improvements is to work with your survey partner to obtain more detailed data, ideally at every whole-number percentile level from 1 to 99. At the very least, your survey partner should be able to provide this information based on their client population, and they may also be willing and able to provide this data based on national data obtained from *hospitalcompare.gov*. Either way, only when you receive percentiles at each level can you accurately plot where your organization is at.

Now all of this discussion about the best way to get detailed percentile data to apply to data that has been downloaded from your survey partner assumes we're talking about percentiles related to a relatively small number of questions or composites. However, the insatiable thirst for percentiles that apply to more and more dimensions of the data (by question and specialty, or by question and hospital/care setting type) gets very tricky very quickly. To put it another way, if you are focused on quarterly performance of your physician

The Display and Use of Data

communication composite, it is pretty easy to pull your score and then look up the value in a table provided by your survey partner to find the percentile. However, to obtain percentiles electronically at every level of analysis (question, specialty, DRG, hospital/care setting type, etc.) and then to marry that to every level of analysis in your internal system is very challenging.

Why is this so challenging? Databases and reporting/visualization tools are leveraged to link and map data all the time. Isn't this just another linking/mapping exercise? Well, not quite. These tools facilitate linking dimensions well, but they are not generally equipped to enable linking aggregations and calculations to tables of benchmarks.

Dimensions are characteristics (or fields) like hospital, physician identifier, patient medical record number, and so on. Aggregations and calculations are counts, averages, sums, and other computations that result in things like average survey response, total number of patients, length of stay, and so on.

For CMS or your survey vendor to calculate the percentile on the fly, as we've already said, it is very easy. Just as there is a database function for calculating averages, there is also one for calculating percentile rank. Since CMS and your survey partner's data contain a population of survey responses beyond your single organization, percentiles are simply another calculation. However, when you've imported just your organization's data into an internal database, and you have a table of published percentiles to map in to that data set, you will have to calculate the average survey response (by whatever dimension is selected by the user, such as a particular question and DRG) and then take that output and attempt to link it to the range of averages that fall into each percentile provided. That kind of simultaneous aggregate-and-link process, though not impossible, is very challenging to do in report/visualization tools.

One solution to this challenge is to precalculate in the database all the aggregations (average scores) at every desired level of dimensionality (e.g., question, specialty, DRG) and then do the linking. This approach can work for static reporting tools but doesn't work well for tools that are more ad hoc in nature, meaning the end user drives the analysis by selecting the dimensions he or she wants to analyze, filtering, and drilling down on data dynamically.

If you didn't follow any of this, the bottom line is that insisting on having percentiles attached at every level of analysis (or even just multiple levels of analysis) in your internal patient experience data will add much complexity and difficulty to the work, without a commensurate gain. As mentioned previously, it is much better to use published percentiles from CMS or your survey partner to set goals and then display progress against your goals in your internal reports and dashboards.

Composites

Composite scores in the world of patient experience data are combinations of multiple survey questions that pertain to a particular theme. For example, the Physician Communication Composite consists of the following questions:

1. During this hospital stay, how often did doctors treat you with courtesy and respect?

2. During this hospital stay, how often did doctors listen carefully to you?

3. During this hospital stay, how often did doctors explain things in a way you could understand?

Each of those individual questions are measured on a 4-point scale (Never/Sometimes/Usually/Always) and then the composite score is calculated as an aggregation of those. The way the composite is aggregated, however, may surprise you. It is actually (using the official CMS calculation) calculated as an average of the average scores of each question. Your math teacher taught you that taking the average of averages is usually a no-no because when the populations (denominators) of the individual averages don't match, your results will be skewed. For example, let's say we have the following surveys (Yes/No indicates a top-box score), and for some reason the question about doctors explaining things was left blank more often than the others:

Survey	Courtesy/Respect	Listen	Explain
1	Yes	Yes	Yes
2	Yes	No	
3	No	No	
4	Yes	No	Yes
5	No	Yes	
6	No	Yes	Yes
Avg	50% Top-Box	50% Top-Box	100% Top-Box

The composite score in this case is (0.5 + 0.5 + 1)/3 or 67% top-box. The "Explain" question is pulling the whole composite score up more significantly than its population justifies.

In large populations, any abnormalities from missed survey questions will balance out, so averaging averages is less of a concern, but if you have a voice in your math conscience that is nagging you, you aren't crazy. In addition, like mapping percentiles instead of calculating them as discussed above, reporting/visualization tools can have trouble with averaging averages as well, so don't be surprised if it takes your analyst or developer a little longer to get composites to calculate properly.

Transparency

We've spent a lot of time talking about percentiles, because we've observed a significant (and often excessive) focus on them everywhere we go. But there are several other important things to consider when determining how to display and use data in your organization. The first is the importance of transparency.

When we talk about transparency of patient experience data, it's helpful to think about it in terms of two extremes. The first extreme is the no-transparency approach: Lock down patient experience results and don't allow one unit, clinic, or provider to see results for any other unit, clinic, or provider. The philosophy at work here is usually that openly displaying peer data only has the potential to embarrass others, and that isn't the way to bring about positive change. These are professionals who just need to know where they are at, and they will be intrinsically motivated to improve.

The second extreme is the total transparency approach: Make unblinded data available at the unit, clinic, and provider level to everyone in the organization. The reasoning is that a little competition is healthy, and knowing that your performance data is visible to all will give a little (or a lot) of extra incentive to improve. Transparency also helps with accountability, as leaders and peers can hold each other accountable, especially when there are shared goals for patient experience improvement. We tend to lean toward the transparent approach as opposed to the locked-down approach, but you will definitely want to proceed toward transparency with caution. We have found that there is a good progression that organizations can use to help prepare providers in particular for full transparency. Pay close attention to the following considerations:

- Make sure your data is accurate. Start with a small scope of data (not a small amount—see the next bullet point—but a limited number of units and a limited number of questions), so you can ensure accuracy before rolling out the data. If you take performance data to physicians and leaders and it is incorrect, it will be very difficult to get them back on your side.

- Ensure you have a sufficient sample size. We tend to shoot for 30–40 surveys per whatever period you are looking at before sharing a new detail level of patient experience performance data. For example, to show provider-level data, hide any providers with fewer than 35 survey responses. Use a three- or six-month average if necessary to get a sufficient sample size.

- Take an incremental approach. Show detailed performance data (i.e., at the unit and provider level), but make it blinded at first so providers and leaders can see how they rank against their peers and other units before that information is open to everyone. From there, show it at the group level unblinded, but keep the provider names blinded. Then, show the providers their data individually. Finally, show the provider-level data internally.

- Focus on improvement. It's hard to argue with getting better on behalf of our patients, so pursue an approach of data transparency for the purposes of improvement as opposed to punishment. Highlight high-performing units and providers, and look for ways to help everyone learn from their successes.

- Communicate your plans clearly. The worst thing you can do is surprise people with public performance data. Instead, communicate the plan for transparency, the timeline, and most importantly of all, the purpose. You have to sell the vision and why this is best for patients if you want to get everyone on board with improvement.

The industry is moving toward greater transparency in quality and patient experience data, so it's best to get your organization used to transparency while it's among friends. But you will want to take a very measured approach in doing so. As one of our favorite physicians said, "If you're going to go naked, you might as well be buff!"

Enterprise Data Warehouse

Earlier in this chapter, we discussed three things to consider before making the decision to direct leaders and physicians in your organization to reports

Chapter 8

on your survey partner's website. With your survey partner's website, there will be limited integration with other key data from your organization, your constituents will have to remember yet another login to yet another website, and they will have to work with nonstandard reporting and visualization functionality. You will not have these issues, however, if you employ a properly designed and well-governed enterprise data warehouse (EDW).

An EDW is a database in which key data from across an organization is standardized, integrated, and enhanced to gain new and better insights, and ultimately drive improved decision-making—or in healthcare terms, better and more efficient care. In a healthcare EDW, you might integrate your patient experience data with quality, operational, and financial data, which would allow you to not only see your performance in those different areas on the same scorecard but also to look for correlations between the different areas to help determine why your scores are what they are, or perhaps gain understanding into the implications of patient experience improvements to performance in other areas.

We are strong advocates of developing an EDW because an EDW allows you to control your destiny as it relates to how you want to see your patient experience data as opposed to being dependent on an outside vendor with all of the competing requests and priorities a vendor has to entertain. If you want to see how your patient experience scores fluctuate according to your daily volumes, or staffing levels, or even local weather, with an internally developed EDW where you can influence the team's priorities, you can do all of those things.

Another benefit of an EDW, aside from being an internal resource that doesn't require maintaining a separate username and password, is that the central analytics environment facilitates standardization of not only metric and data element definitions but also of the tools used to access and visualize the data. It is much more efficient for the organization and easier for end users to have a single set of tools that cover the major needs—ad hoc querying of data, generating static reports, and interactive visualization (dashboards)—than having to learn a new tool for every different data subject (like patient experience data).

All of this isn't to say developing an EDW is easy. It isn't. It requires a talented and driven development team, strong leadership support, and unwavering dedication to pragmatic and end user–focused guiding principles. A successful EDW effort is truly an enterprise effort, not just one leader's pet project in a single area. If any of the above isn't present, trying to force an internal reporting solution for patient experience data may be more hassle than it is worth, and the best approach may be to rely on your survey partner for reporting. However, if you are able to leverage a strong EDW offering at your organization, you will ultimately be far better off in your analytics capabilities.

Ultimately, the key thing to remember when it comes to patient experience data is this: Let the data work for you, but don't become bogged down in the data. Use the data to see how you are performing, then set goals and get on the road to improvement.

References

Centers for Medicare & Medicaid Services. (2016). Retrieved June 27, 2016, from *www.hcahpsonline.org/Files/April-May_2016_Summary%20Analyses_Pctls.pdf*

Section 5
Methods

Chapter 9
Communication Counts

Establishing connections and beginning collaborative improvement requires many things. We've talked about the projection of patient and family voices and being mindful of employee engagement and physician satisfaction as essential elements to establishing those connections. Setting up for success in collaborative improvement requires strategy regarding leadership, executive sponsorship, structure, and support. Building an in-depth knowledge of the data and its limitations, as well as helping maximize its value and use in the organization, is essential to collaborative improvement. Once these elements are in place, you can focus on key areas for the organization. It's rare that I work with an organization where communication is not an area of focus in one way, shape, or form. Let's look at some of those best practices in improving communication.

Chapter 9

Key Care Practices Across the Continuum

What do you notice about this bowl of M&M's?

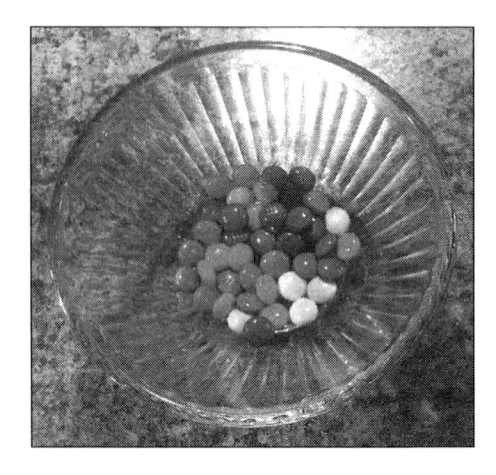

"It's colorful." Yes.

"Lots of primary colors." Yes.

"Someone's been eating some of them." Yes.

What's the significance of this bowl of M&M's to communication and patient experience? Well, believe it or not, notorious rock band Van Halen had a contract rider demanding a bowl of M&M's backstage—with all of the brown M&M's removed. Contrary to popular belief at the time, it wasn't because they were simply rock divas; they were operations masters. The "M&M clause," buried in the middle of critical technical specifications of their contract, was their canary in the coal mine. The presence or absence of brown M&M's was a way to quickly assess if people were paying attention to every word of their contract. The idea was that if this small, less significant detail was missed, larger safety details may have also been missed. This was a big deal when they were going into different markets with more elaborate setup and shows than had been done quite that way before (Ganz, 2012; Jones, 2014).

Communication Counts

I honestly believe, after all of my work in the area of patient experience and communications, there is a similar phenomenon in the connection between courtesy and respect, listening carefully, and explaining things in a way that can be understood. Consider this example.

I was sick with a respiratory issue, so I made an appointment at my clinic; not with my provider, but for the first available time so it wouldn't interrupt my day. I came in with my 2-year-old son, and we got roomed pretty quickly. But that's when things slowed to a crawl. I riffled through my purse and found some snacks. We read every automotive magazine that they had.

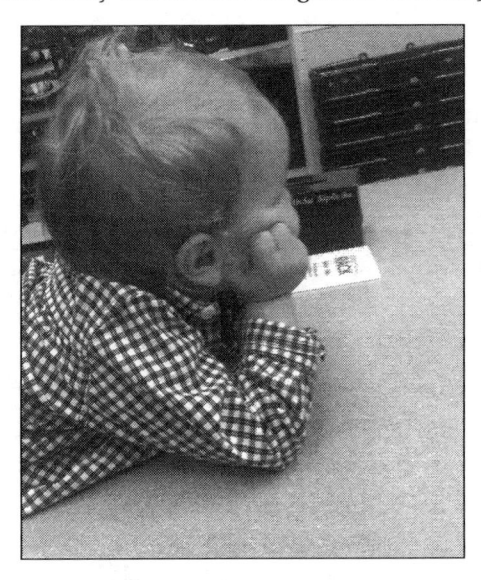

By the time the physician came in, I had spent a total of 63 minutes waiting in a room with a 2-year-old boy! If you know anything about a longer-than-expected wait with a toddler, you know what kind of stress I was dealing with! I thought I had done a really good job, so I was just looking for some acknowledgment of the wait.

When the physician walked in, he didn't even acknowledge it. It wasn't just his lack of an apology for being late, but he offered no pleasantries of any kind. There were a lot of even not-so-direct ways that this physician could

Chapter 9

have let me know that he appreciated what I had been through. But he didn't exhibit one bit of empathy.

Here's the link back to the basics and the brown M&M's: The physician I saw, who showed no empathy for my hour-plus-long wait with a toddler, didn't show me any courtesy or respect. Consequently, as I shared why I was there and what I was concerned about, I didn't feel like he listened carefully to me. My perception was that he thought I was there seeking antibiotics, when I really just wanted to know if I was healthy enough to keep going in and out of patients' rooms shadowing and coaching care team members. Later, I remembered that I didn't ask about something at the appointment, and I realized that we hadn't been communicating at all. I didn't feel like I was being heard, and I certainly didn't feel like he could explain things in a way that I could try to understand.

The reality is that communication counts. It makes a difference if patients feel heard and understood, as well as how they can then understand their providers.

At the Heart of It All: Empathy

One of my first tasks as a director of patient experience was to present to a group of hospitalists about physician communication and share a few key strategies for them to focus on for improvement. I was new to my role and new to the field. Specifically, I'd been instructed to talk to the doctors about empathy and teach back. The general understanding was that if they just did those two things, then all of our problems would be solved! How naive! But anyway, out I went in the hospital to present to the hospitalists over their lunch meeting.

As a social worker, I took classes and wrote papers on empathy, but I knew I needed to be careful when trying to talk to a group of physicians about empathy. I chose my words very carefully as I broached the subject. I said, "Now, it's not for a minute that I don't think you *have* empathy. I believe that you entered healthcare and this profession because you came from a place of wanting to help people and make a difference. You're bright, talented people who could have chosen a different field besides medicine. I believe that the fact that you chose this came from a place of empathy and caring about the health of the patients you serve. The challenge is for you to *consistently demonstrate* that empathy to the patients and families that you care for each day."

Before I knew it, a hand shot up in the back of the room. One of the hospitalists, Dr. Khan, said, "It's like my wife!" I paused, a little unsure of where this was headed and said, "Okay … tell me more."

He continued, "Well, do I love her, yes. But if you asked her on a survey about whether or not I consistently do things that demonstrate that to her, I'm not so sure she'd check 'Always!'" Everyone laughed, and I breathed a sigh of relief. Dr. Khan illustrated my point exactly! We're not talking about whether you *have* empathy or feel it for patients and their families; the challenge is to *demonstrate* it consistently so that they can perceive it.

Ever since that meeting, I always preface my comments about empathy whenever I'm speaking to any group with this distinction that it's not about *having* but *demonstrating* empathy to patients and families. I find that this helps to decrease any would-be defensiveness among those present. Besides, I believe it. In the coaching that I've done with hundreds of care team members, it's not that I'm trying to help teach them to have empathy. More often, what I'm encouraging them to do is to demonstrate the empathy that they are feeling. I'll have to say things like "I know you're thinking it, just say it." I can't tell you how many times I'll be shadowing a caregiver and we'll leave the room and out in the hall, they'll say something to me like, "Man, that guy has had a rough go of it. He's been in and out of here too many times to count in the last few months. He's feeling really crummy and I wish we could get him some answers." In those moments, I challenge the care team member to share

Chapter 9

with the patient just what was shared with me! It's okay to say that to the patient and to really let him or her know that you can put yourself in someone else's shoes and try to see it through his or her eyes.

French author Marcel Proust wrote: "The real voyage of discovery consists not in seeking new landscapes, but in having new eyes."

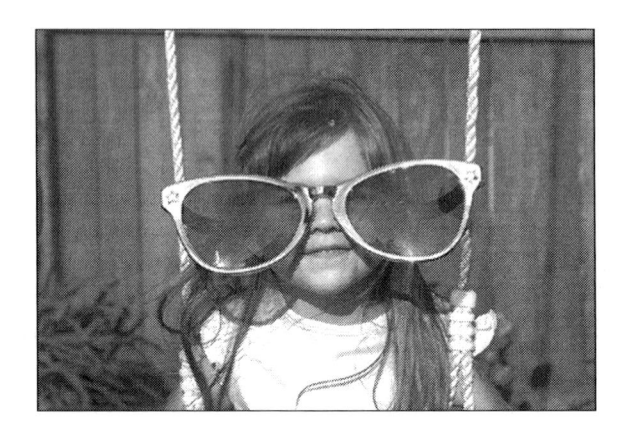

One of my favorite authors is Brené Brown. It's not just because she's a social worker—although that definitely raises the cool factor in my mind—but she has such a great sense of humor and is just plain awesome at defining and explaining things. She's done several TED Talks and authored plenty of books on topics such as courage, vulnerability, authenticity, shame, and empathy (Brown, 2012, 2010, 2007).

It was through Brené that I first heard of the work of Theresa Wiseman, a nursing scholar who has also looked extensively at the topic of empathy. Wiseman talks about the four essential components of empathy (1996):

1. Perspective taking—able to see the world as others see it

2. Staying out of judgment

3. Recognizing emotion in others—understanding another person's feelings

4. Being able to respond to that—communicate your understanding of another person's feelings

Sometimes I think we are doing well to achieve #1, perspective taking. Quite honestly, in most of the work that I do with care teams around the country, often our focus is just getting them to stop, breathe, and be able to tap into that empathy by just seeing the situation from their patient's perspective. Sometimes that's all we can do—get them to see it from their patients' eyes. I see the real work beginning when we can focus on #2–#4. The staying out of judgment is so very hard for so many of us. I find it to be especially challenging for those who have been in this industry for a while. When they are seeing the cardiac/chest pain, sepsis, miscarriage, or trauma for the first time, their empathy and lack of judgment is stronger than when they've seen it for the sixth time … this week!

One of the best tools that I have for staff is a YouTube video by Brené Brown. In it, she so creatively and humorously talks poignantly about the subject. One of the key learnings and challenges that I have taken from her in this is the idea of not "silver-lining it." She talks about how one of our natural reactions when someone tells us something hard or difficult is to try to put the silver lining around it and try to make it better. She points out that rarely does an empathic response begin with "at least," and she shares some examples:

- "I had a miscarriage." … "At least you know you can get pregnant."

- "I think my marriage is falling apart." … "At least you're married."

- "John is getting kicked out of school." … "At least Sarah is an A student."

Brown talks about how natural it is for each of us to try to do this after someone shares something painful with us. After hearing this, I've been convinced of how many times the silver lining is my natural reaction, to try to make it better and give the person perspective on how it could be worse by pointing out the positive. A colleague and I were teaching a workshop together, and we'd been discussing this nuance to empathy with an interdisciplinary team. Later that night, my colleague received a text from a dear friend who was going through a divorce. She said that her first reaction was to respond with something to try to cheer the friend up and help put a silver lining on it. What she did instead was delete her first text response and typed something more on the lines of "Boy, that's tough. I'm sorry. I am so glad you told me, and I'm here for you."

According to Brown, one of the best things we can do when someone shares something painful is to respond with: "Phew, I don't even know what to say … I'm just so glad you told me" (2013). Brown points out that what fuels empathy is *connection*. I feel blessed to have some very close friends with whom we can challenge one another and support each other through the hard parts of life. Even as I write this, I can hear one of them saying throughout countless experiences: "Wow, that's a lot. I'm so glad you told me." It's like she has Brown's playbook memorized!

One of the best resources for sharing about empathy is the YouTube video released by the Cleveland Clinic in 2013 entitled "Empathy: The Human Connection to Patient Care" available at: *www.youtube.com/watch?v=cD-DWvj_q-o8At* (Cleveland Clinic, 2013). As of this writing, there are over 2.7 million hits, and I'm pretty sure I'm singlehandedly responsible for at least a couple hundred of them. If you haven't seen the video, you really should. It begins with this quote: "Could a greater miracle take place than for us to look through each other's eyes for an instant?" —Henry David Thoreau

The general premise is showing patients, family members, and staff going throughout their interactions with little thought bubbles above their heads about what they are thinking—both happy and sad thoughts, what they are excited about as well as what they are worried about. It beautifully illustrates the cacophony of energy and emotions that are coursing through each clinic, hospital, long-term care facility, or home health interaction each day.

Sometimes we forget that our patients' lives don't stop when they come to us for care. The same thing is true for our staff.

I shared this with an interdisciplinary team of emergency room doctors, nurses, techs, and social workers, and asked if they felt like it would be applicable to use with their colleagues. As the video concluded, with tears streaming down their cheeks, I got some enthusiastic nods (yes), even though no one could quite speak up, as they were so choked up.

The reason that I like to use that video is not just because it's so well done, but because it helps to illustrate another key point, in addition to empathy: why this is all so hard. When we talk about listening carefully, showing courtesy and respect, and explaining things well—that just sounds easy. The reality is that each and every day we all come to work and there's an invisible bubble above our heads. There's the landscape and the backdrop of our lives outside of that moment that shapes who we are and how we are able to show up to each interaction that day. This is absolutely true for each patient and family member who we encounter throughout that day. I find that it helps to acknowledge that what we're talking about in terms of key communication practices are not, in and of themselves, difficult. What makes them difficult are two things: who we are, and who we're caring for and interacting with in that moment.

Who we are encompasses everything going on for us before we got there and the things we're worried or excited about when we leave. Both of these can lead to us being distracted and having a hard time truly being present for our patients. Because of these things going on in our own lives—the good and the bad—it makes it even more difficult to truly engage and demonstrate empathy. Think about it: If I'm having a great day, I just got engaged over the weekend, and my head is swimming with the details of upcoming wedding and planning frenzy, it may be hard for me to step out of that enough to see my patient. To truly empathize with where they are, just receiving a critical diagnosis or learning that the only solution involves an amputation or more chemotherapy, etc., is hard. For some staff, they don't want to squelch their own joy to step back and truly imagine what their patients are enduring at that moment. For others, they're dealing with a lot at home—a sick child with multiple health concerns, and the call today confirmed that the next step is to discuss palliative care. Imagine the unmistakable grief for that parent, a nurse, who then has to go in and be truly present with a soon-to-be mom who just saw a heartbeat on her ultrasound for the first time.

These are tough situations, and it's why everything we're talking about in terms of communication sounds simple, but is anything but that. If we don't take into account and address the issues of resiliency needed to support our physicians and care team members, we're on a collision course that can only lead to burnout.

Three Good Things

Given this increasing propensity toward burnout, one of the key strategies to be mindful of with patient experience, is resiliency for staff and physicians. Traditionally, resiliency has been understood as an individual's ability to overcome adversity and continue his or her normal development. However, in his work with resilience across cultures, Dr. Michael Ungar suggests that resilience may be better understood:

> *In the context of exposure to significant adversity, whether psychological, environmental, or both, resilience is both the capacity of individuals to navigate their way to health-sustaining resources, including opportunities to experience feelings of well-being, and a condition of the individual's family, community and culture to provide these health resources and experiences in culturally meaningful ways (2008).*

Consider this study from *Business Insider*. Using data from the Occupational Information Network (O*NET), a U.S. Department of Labor database full of detailed information on jobs, researchers found the 29 professions you should avoid if you really don't like stress. O*NET assigns a "stress tolerance" score (0–100)—which measures how frequently workers must accept criticism and deal effectively with high stress on the job—for each of the almost 900 jobs in its database. A lower rating signals less stress; a higher rating signals more. Of the 29 jobs with a stress tolerance rating of 94 or greater, 19 of them are in healthcare. I won't list them all here, but suffice it to say nurses are all over this list, as are various specialties of physicians. And, even a few roles you may not have thought of: phlebotomists, healthcare social workers, and telephone operators all made the list. Bottom line is that it's stressful to work in healthcare, in particular in frontline roles (Smith, 2016).

This is why building resiliency among the care team is paramount. There's a rather amazingly simple antidote for this gaining some traction across the globe, but also among the care team in healthcare. Dr. Martin Seligman, a founding father of positive psychology, focused on changing from the traditional "disease model" of psychology, which focuses on how to relieve suffering and more on how to enhance well-being (Seligman, 2005). Seligman suggests the "What-Went-Well Exercise" also known as the "Three Blessings." He and his team at the University of Pennsylvania's Positive Psychology Center have validated these in experiments they have been conducting since 2001 studying changes in subjects' life satisfaction and depression levels (Sexton, 2014).

Seligman's empirically tested antidote:

> *Every night for the next week, set aside 10 minutes before you go to sleep. Write down three things that went well today and why they went well. You may use a journal or your computer to write about the events, but it is important that you have a physical record of what you wrote. The three things need not be earthshaking in importance ("My husband picked up my favorite ice cream for dessert on the way home from work today"), but they can be important ("My sister just gave birth to a healthy baby boy").*

Next to each positive event, answer the question "Why did this happen?" For example, if you wrote that your husband picked up ice cream, write "because my husband is really thoughtful sometimes" or "because I remembered to call him from work and remind him to stop by the grocery store." Or if you wrote, "My sister just gave birth to a healthy baby boy," you might pick as the cause, "She did everything right during her pregnancy." (Seligman, 2012)

There are apps out there to help you with this, in case you're wondering! I personally have been experimenting with one simply called "Gratitude!" For those who practice these exercises for two weeks or more, Seligman promises that we'll be "less depressed, happier, and addicted to this exercise six months from now" (Sexton, 2014; Seligman, 2012; Popova, n.d.).

In our work, we've had the opportunity to participate in projects related to promoting resiliency. With one group, the focus was with hospitalists and surgeons. They were given a pre- and post-test to measure resiliency and burnout (Maslach Burnout Inventory and The Brief Resiliency Scale). In between the tests, for five months, they would engage in a Three Good Things activity and journal it each day. When comparing those who did the Three Good Things activity from the pre- to post-surveys, both surgeons and hospitalists showed a decrease in burnout rate.

I'm completely taken with this simple notion that gratitude can change things—in our own lives and in the lives of others. This is of paramount importance in enabling our care team members—as they face difficult situations every day—to remain focused and be mindful and present with their patients. It is imperative that the team supporting and leading this improvement work in patient experience be mindful and focused on this key variable as well.

Fig. 9.1: Three Good Things Poster

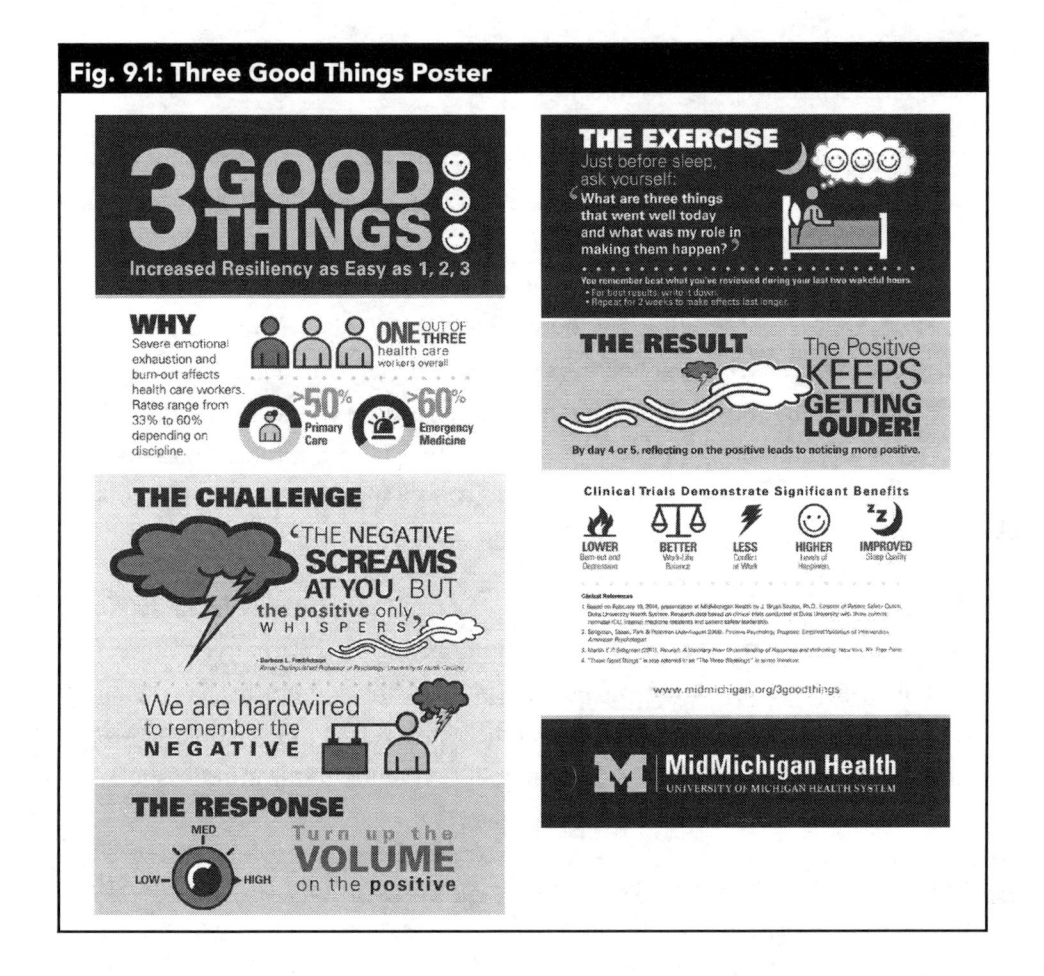

Mindfulness

Empathy, compassion, courtesy, respect, listening carefully, and giving good explanations all have one thing in common: mindfulness. To be truly present with another person, we have to be mindful. Have you ever talked to someone on the phone, but you could tell that they were multitasking? I've been guilty of this myself, and I try to step away from the computer if I am on a call, lest I get distracted or am tempted to multitask a bit. This can happen in person, too. We can be with someone and be present physically but not mentally and certainly not emotionally.

Have you ever been reading a children's story aloud and read the words but not followed the context? Sometimes, late at night when I'm putting my kids to bed, I can read the words to *One Fish, Two Fish, Red Fish, Blue Fish* (the longest Dr. Seuss book ever in my opinion), but I have made several page turns without really "reading" it to my kids. I often wish there was a recorder going and wonder what my voice sounded like when this phase-out happens and I'm thinking about something else while reading the words aloud. Now, that's not a proud momma moment to admit that I am multitasking while reading bedtime stories. It's not something that happens often, and when it happens, I try to catch myself and be more mindful.

Maybe something similar has happened to you. Have you ever been driving somewhere and arrived at your destination only to realize that you didn't remember much about your journey? Or been eating something like a snack bar and looked down and realized that all that is left is the wrapper in your hand? These are common examples of going on autopilot or mindlessness, and are not uncommon in our busy lives today.

It's easy to lose the moment as we juggle work, home, family, finances, stress, and relationships. This can happen to caregivers, too. Consider when they are doing a task for the 10th time that day and the 30th time that week and can be on autopilot. Taking the time to realize that while it may be the 100th time you've done a computerized tomography scan, it may be the first time this patient has ever had one.

To really exhibit empathy and compassion and to communicate with care, we need to be mindfully present. What is mindfulness? According to Jon Kabat Zinn, professor of medicine emeritus and creator of the Stress Reduction Clinic and the Center for Mindfulness in Medicine, Health Care, and Society at the University of Massachusetts Medical School: "Mindfulness means paying attention in a particular way, on purpose, in the present moment, non-judgmentally" (Kabat-Zinn and Nhat Hanh, 2013).

Juliet Adams, founder of *Mindfulnet.org* and director of A Head for Work writes of the ABCs of Mindfulness:

- A is for awareness—becoming more aware of what you are thinking and doing—what's going on in your mind and body.

- B is for "just being" with your experience—avoiding the tendency to respond on autopilot and feed into problems by creating your own story.

- C is for seeing things and responding more wisely—by creating a gap between the experience and our reaction to it, we can make better choices.

Being present for our patients and families provides individualized care and helps to ease their anxiety. It is when we are fully present that we are truly able to convey to them that we are listening carefully. I believe it's only with mindful presence that empathy can truly be demonstrated such that it is perceived (Mindfulnet.org, n.d.).

Whenever I'm asked to speak about empathy and communication, I always end up talking about mindfulness. There was one nurse who I worked with at United Hospital who said, "Before I enter each patient's room, I pause at the doorway, close my eyes, and count to 10. This helps clear my mind and focus on the patient at hand."

Now, when I've shared that with some nurses, they say, "Yeah, right, I don't have time to count to 10." And that's fine, but I encourage them to at least take one big cleansing breath before they enter patients' rooms. One night I was shadowing with a nurse who literally ran down the hallway. I was worried that she was doing this because I was there. I commented that it must be a particularly busy evening because she ran most of the time between the med room and patients' rooms, etc. The nurse assured me that that was her usual pace every evening. Anyway, at the end of my time with this nurse, one of the things I coached her on was knocking before she entered patients' rooms and using that moment to take a breath herself. This woman's anxiety had to be off the charts, and she was carrying that with her into each and every patient's room like a Tasmanian devil. Think about what a different presence it would create if she could pause and breathe before she entered her patients' rooms.

We've covered various communication aspects and discussed how they are key to improvement across the continuum. There are building blocks from courtesy and respect to listening carefully to explaining things well. Underneath it all, though, we must start with a bedrock of empathy, which requires building on the skills of both mindfulness and resiliency.

References

Brown, B. (2012). *Daring greatly: How the courage to be vulnerable transforms the way we live, love, parent, and lead.* New York, NY: Gotham Books.

Brown, B. (2010). *The Gifts of Imperfection: Let go of who you think you're supposed to be and embrace who you are.* Center City, MN: Hazelden.

Brown, B. (2007). *I Thought It Was Just Me: Women reclaiming power and courage in a culture of shame.* New York, NY: Gotham Books.

Cleveland Clinic. (2013). *Empathy: The human connection to patient care* [video file]. Retrieved June 27, 2016, from *www.youtube.com/watch?v=cDDWvj_q-o8At*

Ganz, J. (2012). The truth about Van Halen and those brown M&M's. Retrieved June 27, 2016, from *www.npr.org/sections/therecord/2012/02/14/146880432/the-truth-about-van-halen-and-those-brown-m-ms*

Jones, S. (2014). No brown M&M's: What Van Halen's insane contract clause teaches entrepreneurs. Retrieved June 27, 2016, from *www.entrepreneur.com/article/232420*

Kabat-Zinn, J., and Nhat Hanh, T. (2013). *Full Catastrophe Living (revised edition): Using the wisdom of your body and mind to face stress, pain, and illness.* United States: Bantam Books.

Mindfulnet.org. (n.d.). What is mindfulness? Retrieved June 27, 2016, from *www.mindfulnet.org/page2.htm*

Popova, M. (n.d.). A simple exercise to increase well-being and lower depression from Martin Seligman, founding father of positive psychology. Retrieved June 27, 2016, from *www.brainpickings.org/2014/02/18/martin-seligman-gratitude-visit-three-blessings/*

Roth, B. (2016). Three easy ways to find your resilience. Retrieved June 27, 2016, from *https://today.duke.edu/2016/02/resilience*

Seligman, M. E., Steen, T. A., Park, N., & Peterson, C. (2005). Positive psychology progress: Empirical validation of interventions. [Abstract]. *Am Psychol.*, 60(5), 410–21.

Seligman, M. E. (2012). *Flourish: A visionary new understanding of happiness and well-being.* New York, NY: Free Press.

Sexton, J. B. (2014). Research data based on clinical trials conducted at Duke University with three cohorts: neonatal ICU, internal medicine residents and patient safety leadership. Presentation at MidMichigan Health in February, 2014.

Smith, J. (2016). 29 jobs to avoid if you hate feeling stressed. Retrieved June 27, 2016, from *www.businessinsider.com/jobs-to-avoid-if-you-dont-like-stress-2016-6*

TexasChildrensVideo. (2012). Dr. J. Bryan Sexton—Three good things [video file]. Retrieved June 27, 2016, from *www.youtube.com/watch?v=hZ4aT_RVHCs*

The RSA. (2013). Brené Brown on empathy [video file]. Retrieved June 27, 2016, from *www.youtube.com/watch?v=1Evwgu369Jw*

Ungar, M. (2011). The social ecology of resilience: Addressing contextual and cultural ambiguity of a nascent construct. *American Journal of Orthopsychiatry, 81,* 1–17.

Ungar, M. (2008). Resilience across cultures. *British Journal of Social Work, 38,* 218–35.

Wiseman, T. (1996). A concept analysis of empathy. *Journal of Advanced Nursing,* 23(6), 1162–1167.

Chapter 10
Spectrum of Strategies

We've looked at how important communication is to achieving the goals of collaborative improvement. Now let's take a look at some specific strategies to employ to reach these goals.

I was communicating with a director of patient relations recently who wrote: "Things are busy as ever. I keep hoping our patient experience work will eventually cut down our complaints/grievances." Whether it's related to complaints and grievances or the scores on the surveys themselves, I still hear plenty of people relying on hope as their strategy. Having a focused plan of how to approach improvement can help take away the guessing, finger-crossing, and silent prayers to help achieve your goals.

Over the years, I have had the opportunity to collaborate with high performers in communication—both in the inpatient/HCAHPS realm and also in the outpatient/CG-CAHPS realm, as well as the emergency department/ED-PEC or ED CAHPS sphere. While some of the strategies that they employ may be slightly different, here are some best practices that have worked for the high performers time and again:

- Take a data-driven approach to identify key performance opportunities.
- Focus on improvement one goal at a time.

Chapter 10

- Involve the staff and/or physicians early on in practice changes.

- Observe the patient experience from a patient's entire journey and perspective.

- Recognize that for patients to be happy, you have to have a happy team. Connect the dots between physician satisfaction, employee engagement, and patient experience.

- Recognize that no plan ever goes exactly as intended, and expect that there will be bumps along the road.

- Accept and expect ongoing change as a part of the reality of healthcare and the improvement journey.

- Hold people accountable—make tough decisions when individual behaviors do not match organizational values.

In addition to some of these key drivers of improvement, I've put together a spectrum of strategies to consider in operationalizing and resourcing this within your organization.

Fig. 10.1: Spectrum of Strategies

	Less	More	Most
Projecting the Patient Voice	Sharing comments, awards	Patient & Family Advisory Council	Patients serving on committees
Data & Reporting	Clinic/site/unit level	Physician level	Enterprise Data Warehouse
Goal Setting & Compensation	Identify areas of focus	Internal scorecard	Tied to physician compensation
Service Strategy & Training	Discuss at provider meetings	Develop/adopt a service mnemonic, Video vignettes	Service training, CMEs
Other	Newsletters, Cards, Care boards	Care team coaching, mystery shopping	SWAT Teams, Patient Centered Medical Home

Resource Investment ($/Time) →

Key Strategies for Improvement

How you organize and implement best practices will help determine how successfully you can improve communications across the continuum. It is imperative that you use your data to help focus your strategies and resources in the areas of greatest impact. Here are some examples:

- Projecting the patient voice—Even more so than the numeric values on the patient surveys, the words of the patients themselves resonate deeply with physicians and other caregivers. At a minimum, start by sharing patients' comments and stories. Put together awards, letters, and recognition opportunities when physicians are specifically named in patient comments. Creating a Patient and Family Advisory Council is another amazing way to get really great feedback about various aspects of communication. Ultimately, many organizations then progress to having patients serve on committees alongside physicians and staff.

- Data and reporting—Sharing the survey and other experience data at the unit, site, or clinic level is a starting point. However, being able to customize and pull the data by the provider group, and ultimately the individual provider/staff member, can lead to transformational progress. These data, accompanied by a process leading to full transparency, are key to achieving even greater results. Some organizations are even extending this internal transparency to their websites and making it public. The most sophisticated level of reporting is found in organizations that create an EDW for broader analysis, combining the clinical and experiential metrics.

- Goal setting and compensation—Start by identifying a key area of focus. From there, many organizations have internal scorecards tracking these metrics and the progress toward goals. Increasingly, organizations will tie physician incentives and/or other components of compensation to achievement of patient experience goals.

- Service strategy and training—At minimum, ensure that ongoing discussion of patient experience and improvement is happening at provider meetings. The next level involves developing or adopting a service mnemonic or other mechanism by which the organization decides to organize its content (e.g., AIDET™, RELATE, LEADER) and providing some videos or other vignettes to help illustrate key points in physician communication. Finally, providing service training and creative continuing medical education (CME) events are great ways to reinforce the behaviors and concepts key to improvement in communication.

- Coaching and creativity—Incorporating strategies ranging from something as simple as photo business cards to share when meeting new patients to newsletters focused on communication and patient experience can be helpful. In the inpatient and emergency areas, having physicians and staff write their names on the care board is a step in the right direction. The next level of commitment and resourcing can support you in a physician shadowing or care team coaching program. Many organizations also utilize a concept of SWAT teams (performance improvement–focused groups that can descend upon a unit, clinic, or department) to focus on improvement areas, as well as working toward designations like patient-centered medical home certification in the clinic setting.

Get Creative

One of the things that I think is so fun about working in this field is the ability to be creative. Some of the most creative elements and events that I've been a part of were some of the most memorable for the staff and physicians who participated—and were some of the most fun to facilitate. Here are two of my favorites.

Black Box CME™

With one organization, we were working on improving physician communication. We were focusing on the employed hospitalists from around 10 hospitals of various sizes around the organization. As such, we adapted from a "Black Box CME™" with a local theater company. We'd heard of another healthcare system in the same city that had done a one-actor play from the patient perspective for their physicians. We worked with the theater company and an independent playwright with some unique healthcare experiences of his own to write the play. Further, we worked out an arrangement granting us permission to use that play again.

It was told from the lens of one patient: a middle-aged truck driver who first goes into the clinic for a question about his hip, but while at the appointment, the physician also finds something going on with his heart. The second scene takes place at home in his living room, where he reflects on his visit with

Chapter 10

the doctor from earlier in the day and his anxiety about the surgery to come. The next scene is him right before surgery in the OR, and his thoughts and feelings. The final scene is him in his hospital room recovering. Instead of using it as just one play straight through as the other organization had done, we separated out the acts and used them throughout the evening, with physicians facilitating discussion after each one.

In between the acts, we had various activities that the physicians participated in throughout the theater. One of the activities was a "Medical Jargon Taboo" based on the popular game Taboo™ from the early 1990s. We'd worked with a group of physicians to create a deck of cards that had conditions that they had to commonly explain to patients: atrial fibrillation, hypertension, COPD, etc. Just like in the typical game of Taboo, we had various other terms that physicians may typically use to explain the word, and they couldn't say those. The whole point of the exercise was to help them work on explaining things in a way that patients could understand.

During one of the intermissions, we had one of the clinical psychologists with a lengthy personal medical and surgical history share his experiences with the physicians from his patient perspective. He engaged and challenged the audience using his real experiences and a colorful delivery, and asked some provocative questions of the group—many of whom he knew rather well.

Another intermission activity that really struck me was what we called "Hospitalist Hot Potato." In this activity, teams were given a question for which there could be many answers. The one I remember most vividly was "Please give examples of an empathetic comment you could make to patients." As the potato was passed to them, they had to think of a statement and say it quickly before passing it to the next team of physicians. As we rotated through different groups of physicians, I was left in awe of how many or how few empathetic comments were voiced. In a few groups, the potato was passed a large number of times because they were able to creatively come up with heartfelt empathetic comments on the spot. However, in most groups, the physicians surprisingly came up with only a few. I think this made an impact on many of them as to the importance of empathy and that beyond feeling empathy for your patients, you must communicate it to them and their families.

It was a delightful evening that started with dinner and then moved into the theater, and then was punctuated with other activities in between. We offered it three or four times over several months. This gave ample opportunity for all of the physicians to attend. The medical director for the hospitalists had made this a mandatory activity. Any physicians who were unable to attend had to participate in a makeup activity, such as writing a patient experience newsletter or another patient experience–based project. Participation in the event was tied to their quality goals for the year.

This was memorable to the physicians, and it was so fun to be a part of. So much of the time, I see people downtrodden and nearly depressed, having been beaten over the head about patient experience scores on a survey. I prefer to take a positive, proactive approach and make things more fun! Events like this one reinforced the work that the medical director and patient experience team had been doing all year in their *Communication With Doctors* newsletter and talks that they had been doing at the various groups' meetings. This event wasn't just a flash in the pan or a flavor of the month; it was a culmination of the work from that year and helped to creatively solidify the principles and comments that had been shared. It solidified the organization's commitment to improving the patient experience, and if nothing else, created quite a buzz among hospitalists and their colleagues.

Chapter 10

Simulation: Act Your Way Into a New Way of Being

Another creative aspect of this work is in the field of simulation. Clinical simulation has been around for a while, but it has started to make its way more into communications training as well (Rosen, 2008; Gaba, 2004).

I first learned about simulation as part of some work in positive deviance that we were doing focused on improving pain management and patient experience. According to the Positive Deviance Initiative:

> *Positive deviance is based on the observation that in every community there are certain individuals or groups whose uncommon behaviors and strategies enable them to find better solutions to problems than their peers, while having access to the same resources and facing similar or worse challenges. The positive deviance approach is an asset-based, problem-solving, and community-driven approach that enables the community to discover these successful behaviors and strategies and develop a plan of action to promote their adoption by all concerned. (Aligning Forces for Quality, 2012).*

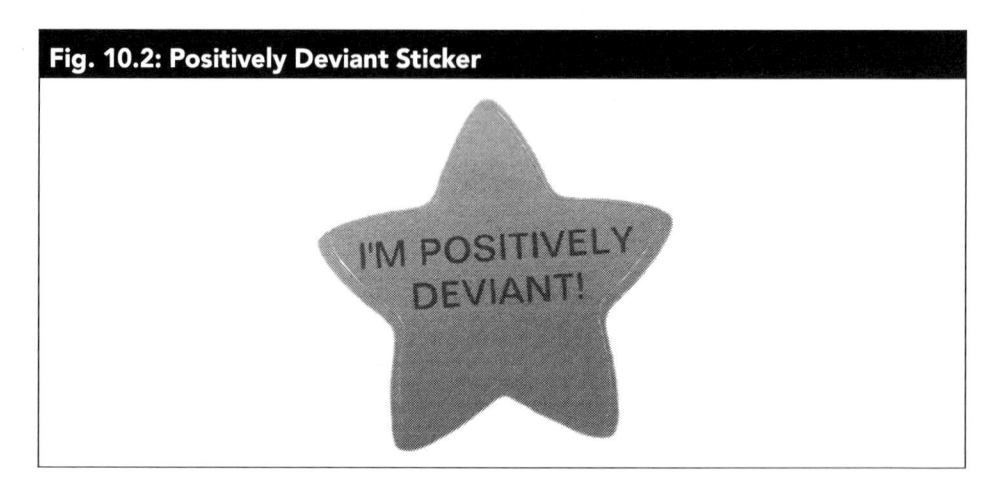

Fig. 10.2: Positively Deviant Sticker

One of the things that I love about positive deviance is that it is so frontline supportive. What I mean is, there's this general belief that the answers lie within. When working with staff-driven frontline teams, we were able to identify key practices that some groups or individuals were using that made a difference in the pain management of their patients, and then we were able to spread those ideas to others. Sounds simple, right? The reality is it's hard and slow work, but very rewarding for those staff engaged in it and very powerful for the organizations participating. Originally used in fighting childhood malnutrition in Vietnam, the principles of positive deviance have been spread into healthcare.

In their book, *Inviting Everyone: Healing Healthcare Through Positive Deviance, 1st Edition*, Arvind Singhal, PhD, Prucia Buscell, and Curt Lindberg, DMan, detail the use of positive deviance (PD) by the Billings Clinic that led to the clinic being able to reduce by 60% its overall rate of potentially deadly MRSA infections. According to the authors,

> At Billings Clinic's 272-bed hospital, healthcare-associated MRSA infections declined 80% house-wide since the positive deviance effort began in late 2006. The number of MRSA infections in the intensive care unit, which served as the PD pilot unit, has dropped to almost zero. In 2005 and 2006, there were 28 total healthcare-associated MRSA infections. In the more than three years since then there have been four ... The hospital engaged frontline employees, those who interact with patients and are likely to be affected by MRSA, asking them how best to address the problem. The efforts were aimed at changing the hospital's culture and everyday behavior (Uken, 2011; Pascale, et. al, 2010).

One of the key principles in this PD work is "A thousand hearings aren't worth one seeing, and a thousand seeings aren't worth one doing." The key idea being that "Seeing trumps hearing, but doing trumps seeing." There are various ways for this to occur. Let's take a look at a few of them.

Chapter 10

A few years ago, my husband had a conference in Florida and I tagged along, just relaxing during the day and meeting up with him at night. When we met up to get ready for the evening's activity, he said, "Well, you're really going to like the event this evening!" And he was right! We visited the University of Central Florida College of Medicine, and were able to tour their facilities. Sounds amazing, right? Well, I completely geeked out when we were able to look at some of their simulation labs. The clinical simulation with all of the high-tech mannequins was really cool. But what I got most excited about (to which my husband told me before we went on that part of the tour, "Now just try not to monopolize the guy by asking so many questions!") was the Communications Simulation Lab.

They had exam rooms set up with video and audio recording capabilities. They used standardized patients (people who were trained actors to come in and pose as patients). The physicians in training were able to learn about communication principles, then actually practice them, and then watch and hear themselves. Additionally, before the standardized patients left the room, they were able to fill out surveys about how they would rate the physician's communication at a computer in the room. Then, when the physicians were able to watch and hear themselves, they also had that data of how those patients perceived them. In case you're wondering, I didn't get all of this information on our tour. I stayed after and talked to the director so as not to embarrass my husband in front of all of his work colleagues!

UCF has a lovely facility, and fortunately, it is not the only medical school using these simulation labs as part of their training. This is becoming increasingly common as part of medical school education. I love that this is how so many medical schools are now training the next generation of physicians (Okuda et al., 2009; Bagnasco et al., 2014; Weller et al., 2012).

This is great for those physicians who are going through their training now or have done so in the last 10 years, as these facilities have started to be used in medical schools across the country. What about those physicians who are

Spectrum of Strategies

already established in their career? What about other care team members who didn't have this as part of their training?

Even in the absence of a sophisticated simulation lab, we have used simulation for communication skills as part of our empathy workshops and communication training sessions with staff and physicians. If you're interested in getting certified as a simulation facilitator, there's more information available from the Society of Simulation in Healthcare and the International Nursing Association for Clinical Simulation and Learning. Also, both of these have listings of places where you can take a class to help build the skills of facilitation. (Visit *www.inacsl.org/i4a/pages/index.cfm?pageid=1 and www.ssih.org/* to learn more.)

I officially took a simulation facilitation course last fall, but that was after years of facilitating communication simulations in patient experience and service culture workshops and trainings. Certification is not necessary to use this effectively with staff and physicians. Some of the training programs are quite clinically focused, and you will have to make your own connections to the use of the modality in communications training. For some, however, the classes may help to inspire greater confidence and build further skills.

When we have used this with a group, it's usually toward the end of a communications workshop. We've usually spent time discussing (hearing) and maybe watching some videos about (seeing) the communication principles. Then, we incorporate simulation as a great way to help solidify and practice (doing) them. We start with some ground rules:

- Have fun
- Uphold your highest level of intelligence
- Go with the flow
- Remain open-minded
- Adopt a posture of learning

Simulation can cause heartburn for some who are anxious being in front of others, so it's important to help make the participants feel more comfortable. These ground rules, together with starting with some volunteers from the audience, help make it more comfortable. The idea is to practice these skills but also have fun in the process and really learn from one another. We encourage participants to "practice at the top of their license." Even in simulation, we expect them to do their best to act with whatever clinical skills they have. Thus, a nurse acts like a nurse and a physician acts like a physician. They are encouraged to bring those skills to the simulation.

It is sometimes helpful to have some simulations developed ahead of time, and I'll share a few basic examples in the following sections below. Those who explore simulation certification will get very involved with the intricacies of making a believable simulation scenario. However, I am also here to say that there are some easy ways to get a general sense of a story and to let the participants run with it. I've also done it where we let the audience and the participants help to design the scenario in the moment.

Often, when doing this, we will ask for someone who is willing to play the patient, as that's the easiest role to play. Once we get the patient up front, we'll ask them what type of patient they'd like to be and what's troubling them. Then, we'll look for a nurse or a physician or an aide to help take care of them, in the clinic, or the hospital, or whatever setting we're working in. Once the volunteer comes up to be that staff person, we'll ask them to help determine whatever other roles they think they need to have there. Sometimes we'll ask the patient if they'd like to have a family member or friend there with them, and then we look for a participant from the audience to be the family member.

The whole idea of simulation is learning in action—both for those participating as well as those observing. It's important for the facilitator to prompt both groups with good questions about what they saw, how it made them feel, and what they would add or do differently. Usually, I will set up the scenario, and

Spectrum of Strategies

let them walk through it for a bit. Then, as the facilitator I will call a timeout or pause, and then ask the participants and the observers some questions. Some examples of the types of questions include trying to get at feelings:

- Asking the participants playing the clinical/care team member roles, "How did you feel that went?"

- Asking the patient, "How did that feel for you?"

- Asking the observers, "What did you see that went well?"

- Depending on what the specific focus areas of the workshop have been, I may ask, "Where did you see AIDET being used? How was compassion displayed? Where did you see empathy? How did they listen carefully?"

- Asking everyone, "What would you add? What would you do differently?"

Here are a few basic scenarios that I have used in group simulation activities:

- Inpatient med-surg unit—certified nursing assistant, patient, spouse, and daughter/son

  - Patient had knee surgery yesterday afternoon.

  - Patient is now on first day postop and this is your first shift with them.

- Emergency room—nurse, patient with cellulitis in the arm, spouse

  - Patient arrived complaining of chest pain and shortness of breath.

  - Patient has just been roomed and you are entering the room for the first time.

  - Spouse is scared and has dementia.

- Clinic—physician, elderly patient, son/daughter bringing elderly parent (patient)

Chapter 10

- Patient has some mobility and ongoing concerns with hip.
- Son/daughter says patient has some memory issues and is wondering if the parent is safe to continue living on his or her own.

Purists would argue with this approach, but I can tell you that in the real world in working with frontline teams who may not want to be at a communications workshop in the first place, engagement is key. Knowing how to get people involved and make it fun, and to not be something that is dreaded, is key to making this simulation technique work for you. Another key is to do this with the right size group. In my experience, the smaller, the better, as it can help to aid in comfort and also participation.

I used this technique recently with a group of supervisors who were going to start rounding patients in the emergency room. Some of them had rounded before, and others hadn't. We'd talked about the key skills and some talking points for doing rounding (hearing), and they'd even watched some videos on it (seeing), but then we gave them a chance to practice it (doing). We divided them into two groups so there were three supervisors in a group with one facilitator. We scheduled this workshop at the right time of day so that one of the pods in the ED was not yet open. We were able to use two actual patient rooms to do some practice. We gave each participant a different scenario, and one by one we worked through each person's scenario. For their scenario, they were the supervisor rounding on the patient, and their colleagues were either the patient and/or family member or friend.

Waiting room

- Younger teenage male, there with his friend.
- Complaining of a toothache and has been waiting for two hours.
- Wants to know how much longer, is worried about missing work.
- Wonders how long till he can get some pain relief.

- Concerned that other people have been arriving after him and have been taken back before him.

Waiting on admission

- Elderly female needs to be admitted through ED with a broken hip and is waiting on surgical consult.
- Patient has her daughter/son in the room with her.
- Patient has a history of dementia.
- Daughter/son have concerns about the amount of pain mom is in and don't like to see her suffering.
- They are not sure who all the caregivers are who have been in and out of their room.
- Want to know when the surgery will be.

Patient "in process"

- The patient is a 50-year-old male with suspected kidney stones waiting on CT results.
- The patient does not like to wait for help.
- His pain is terrible, but he is scared he will get addicted to pain medication.
- Wife is with him and is very anxious and concerned.
- Wondering what's coming next and when they'll know what's happening/what the plan is for his care.

During each scenario, I would stop the group and ask the members about the experience, how it felt, and what they would change or add. We also debriefed it at the end. Each scenario went on for about five to seven minutes. The supervisors talked about how doing this helped them feel more confident

Chapter 10

to then go out and round on real patients. After they had been doing their rounding for a while, we followed that up by doing some care team coaching with them. (We will have more on care team coaching later in this chapter.)

It was a really nice progression that worked well to talk about the principles; see them in action with colleagues; have a safe space to try it out for themselves; then practice on their own for a bit, and follow that with some helpful reinforcement of their strengths and any opportunities.

Simulation can be a very effective method for allowing skills practice of key communication principles. But it's not always for everyone. In one organization, we were designing a training workshop with an interdisciplinary team from the Emergency Department (ED). This facility had an amazing Simulation Lab where it had converted an entire nursing unit into simulation rooms. The lab had all of the high-tech equipment and capabilities to really do a lot with the simulation and training. The staff of the ED had used the Sim Lab quite a bit for their technical training. At the same time as this workshop was about to rollout, all the staff who wanted to work in the mental health-dedicated section of the ED had to go through a 16-hour class that was held over two days in the Sim Lab.

As we were creating this workshop focused on key communication practices for improving the patient and family experience, we talked to an interdisciplinary group of staff, physicians, and leaders to get their input on what should be included and how the content should be delivered. My team, together with the leaders of the department, had always assumed that we'd use the Sim Lab for some/all of the workshop. We thought we'd hold it in that space and then have breakouts for doing the simulation in some of the rooms that were set up for that. But what we heard from the staff, physicians, and supervisors was something very different. We heard things like:

- "ED people hate role-playing. I would avoid this!"
- "We're just 'simmed' out right now …"

Spectrum of Strategies

We discussed this as a group. Many people wanted to have the opportunity for skills practice and definitely saw the value but were concerned about their colleagues' desire and engagement with that modality. Plus, the sessions were going to have about 30 people in them. The group talked about how, really, you have to have everyone participate and rotate through the simulations (like what I was able to do with the supervisors practicing their rounding) to get the full value. The rest of the participants are really just observing their colleagues in action.

Finally, one physician spoke up with a great idea. "What if we wrote a screenplay and filmed it from the patient's perspective? Then the participants would have to watch and find the things that the care team did well, as well as those that could be improved!" Then another physician jumped in: "I have a GoPro and we could strap it to the person's head and film it all!" Thus began the idea.

Two staff physicians and a resident, along with my team and the superb staff from the Sim Lab, sat down and created the first draft of this production. We worked hard to have the nurses and techs and other staff members review and edit the script. They each worked painstakingly to ensure that every person in the scenario exhibited both positive as well as less-than-stellar skills. There wasn't fully scripted text as much as a bulleted outline and some key phrases that they hoped would weave in. Then we picked a day to film it, taking one room of a busy Level 1 Trauma Center out of commission for several hours. The staff and physicians from the interdisciplinary team played themselves. Again, the script was more of an outline, so they completely improv'd it just as they would have in a live simulation. The Sim Lab staff played the simulated patients/embedded actors: the patient and her daughter.

It was amazing! They did a great job and there were some very funny unscripted and also poignant moments that arose from the work. We grouped it into four scenes and used it in the workshops with staff. As one physician told me, "ED people love to see people they know—it's important that staff and physicians play themselves." We gave the participants in the workshop a worksheet, and they were supposed to identify the strengths as well as the opportunities that they saw from a communications perspective and to jot down who (which role) represented them. In between each scene, we would stop to discuss the scene and reflect on what they saw, how that made them feel, and what they would do differently. We also made it a contest. The first round/scene was for practice but after that we had a prize for the person who could identify the most care practices in action—both the strengths and the opportunities. This kept the group engaged.

Looking at the reviews of this workshop, this video "Through the Patients' Eyes" was definitely the highlight for those attending. Later on, there was a provider who I was coaching as follow-up to the workshop. When we were debriefing his personal strengths and opportunities, he asked me if I remembered the video in the workshop, the one shot from the patient's lens. He talked about how even months later that stuck with him, as he'd never seen care from that vantage point before. He himself had never been a patient. Seeing that video helped him see what things look like and may feel like from a patient and family perspective.

At the end of the day, that's what the goal is with all of this: to help connect and engage physicians and staff to be motivated on how they can improve the care they provide. Focusing from the patient and family view is an effective means to help them do this.

No Silver Bullet, But ...

Someone recently ended a post on one of the many patient experience listservs that I frequent with this phrase: "Good luck, and if anyone discovers the silver bullet, do share!" This sentiment is not only true for those working in the field each and every day, but it is also true for the leaders of their organizations as well. Everyone is looking for the silver bullet—a quick fix, something that solves all of the problems, something to make it easier in this work.

The closest thing that I have found to said silver bullet is a combined approach of training supplemented and reinforced by personal, one-on-one shadow coaching. What makes this powerful is the individualized approach. When we talk about improving concepts of courtesy and respect, listening carefully, explaining things in a way that patients and families understand, demonstrating empathy, addressing pain, and engaging in shared decision- making, these are best assessed in the moment and with actual patient encounters.

For most physicians and staff, when they sit in a class and learn about these concepts or are reminded about them, often they say that they don't really know how they do those aspects. I think there's a general personal positive bias that we are better on those aspects than others around us. Let's face it, no one wants to do a bad job of communicating and deliberately disrespecting people. When I have had the opportunity to work one-on-one with care team members, I've seen firsthand the power that this modality can bring.

A word or two about coaching

When an organization is first introducing the concept of shadowing or coaching, it's important to be cognizant of the language used to describe the process. For many, the word "coaching" conjures up performance improvement plans and being "coached out" of the organization. That's entirely the opposite of what this is all about. I've found that a strengths-based approach is not only supportive of the care team but is also a very powerful change agent.

Strengths-based approach

I'm not huge into assessments and personality tests. But there is one that I really believe in: the Clifton StrengthsFinder®. Dr. Donald Clifton is seen as the father of strengths-based psychology, and based on his research he created this assessment tool, leading millions of people around the world to help discover their personal strengths. More than 7 million people have now taken Gallup's StrengthsFinder assessment, and there are resources for readers on how to use this tool with teams and in mapping collective groups' strengths (Rath & Conchie, 2009; Rath, 2007).

What I love about this assessment is that it's just so positive. Shortly before starting our consulting company, I took it for the first time. My partners at the time also took it with me, and together we mapped out our collective team profile, seeing where we had a lot of things in common as well as some areas where strengths were missing. I also did this with several patient experience teams that I have led. I find it to be a very helpful exercise for any team working together. However, I find it to be especially useful when training a group of staff to become coaches. One of the things I like to do when providing a train-the-trainer for coaching is to have the soon-to-be coaches take the StrengthsFinder ahead of the first training session. I find that this gives us a language for where we each shine. It also sets the stage that we are coming from a strengths-based approach when we go out to coach others.

In 2011, Atul Gawande, MD, MPH, a surgeon, public health researcher, and writer for *The New Yorker*, wrote an article in the magazine that highlighted the notion of coaches for physicians. It was such fortuitous timing that the release of this article coincided with the advent of my opportunity to start coaching physicians on communication: As my team embarked on coaching an initial cohort of 75 physicians, we were able to reference this article as a starting point in recruiting participants.

> "We have to keep developing our capabilities and avoid falling behind."
> —Atul Gawande, *The New Yorker* (2011)

It has turned out to be one of the most profound experiences of my career. Observing the physician/patient encounter is such sacred space, and yet it's proven to be an extremely powerful modality for making changes and having lasting impact. I now have had the privilege of coaching more than 300 physicians, physician assistants, nurses, techs, nursing assistants, and the list goes on. Through this experience I have identified some of the keys to success in care team or shadow coaching.

One of the biggest lessons is to partner with those who want to participate. Those who self-select are more engaged and ready to hear, understand, and make lasting changes to improve their current practices. A great way to do this is to present the option to the entire group. Allow physicians and/or other staff to sign up—rarely does every member of the group elect to participate.

Many times, organizations want to use coaching as a way to focus on the low performers, and I really caution them against this as a strategy. There are two reasons for this:

1. Usually there is so much more going on with the low performers that patient experience is the least of your worries.

2. I have seen several organizations achieve great success by simply allowing the high performers or the "always" team to sign up. Then, a few of the "usuallys" will also sign up. All we're trying to do is move the "usuallys" to "always" and ensure some healthy competition.

From strictly a numbers or CAHPS perspective, all you need to do is move the bell-shaped curve to the right. Focusing on the outliers or the "nevers" will not in and of itself get you substantial numerical success.

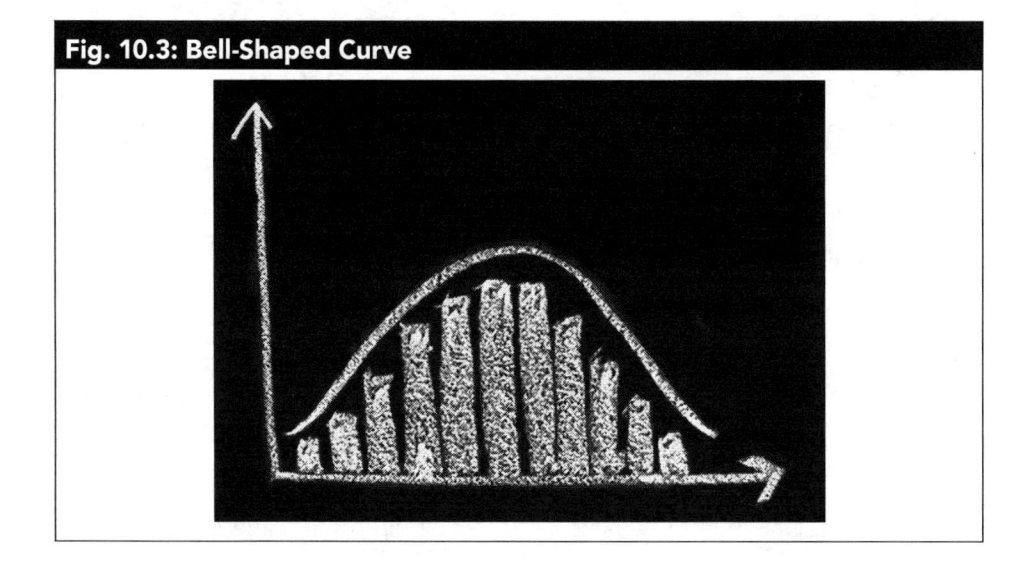

Fig. 10.3: Bell-Shaped Curve

I once had a physician sign up for a coaching session when he was 18 months from retirement. When I asked why he elected to participate, he said, with a bit of emotion in his voice, "I just want to connect with my patients in a better way such that I can help them make life-altering decisions that impact their health and happiness."

Another client, a psychologist, explained her participation when she said, "I received a lot of supervision and feedback during my training, but now that I'm out in my own practice, I'm never sure if I'm really doing a great job or if I could be doing better."

Medical students today go through communications training and participate in simulation labs where standardized patients can rate them on their performances. Hidden cameras and audio recorders also provide instantaneous feedback on their interactions. Unfortunately, many of the older physicians in practice now didn't benefit from these types of experiences as part of their training years ago.

While we can talk about the concepts of showing empathy and incorporating teach back, theories come to life in an observation-and-feedback situation. Physicians and other staff report that this is where they are able to truly understand how to incorporate these aspects effectively into their practices.

I've seen coaching have an immediate impact on practice changes, becoming a positive catalyst for change in an organization. I've rounded with physicians in the morning, made some suggestions, and, later that day, received emails on how those subtle changes produced dramatically different results that afternoon!

One morning I was shadowing with a hospitalist who had been in practice for at least 10 years, so she knew her stuff. After we got done, we sat outside of the ED and debriefed the experience. I talked to her about her many strengths and some of the inconsistencies (things she did some but not all of the time). Then I talked to her about two opportunities I'd witnessed in our time together. One of them was how she explained things, and after she did, how she inquired about her patients' questions. She'd always ask (as most of us do), "Do you have any questions?" To this, the patients responded without critically thinking to the yes/no question, "No."

My challenge to her was to flip this and to use more of an open-ended question by asking, "What questions do you have for me?" I told her that my crazy way of remembering that was thinking of A & W root beer. I always try to remember to change a closed question to an open-ended one by changing the "Any" to "What." That seemed to make sense to her, and we said goodbye as she went off to see her patients for the afternoon. Later that evening, I received an email from her. She was so excited:

"Guess what?! My patients do have questions! All this time I've been going around thinking that I was doing such a great job of explaining things. But this afternoon, I tried what you said and it worked! Just by subtly asking the question differently, it got out more of those questions that they really had for me!"

> *"A small suggestion can go a long way. Many of us physicians have habits we repeat a dozen times a day or more—such as how we greet a patient or how to frame a question. Even a small suggestion that changed the way I ask a common question has already made a positive impact on my care hundreds of times."*
>
> —Physician participant in shadow coaching

To mandate or not to mandate, that is the question

One of the biggest jumps that organizations make is to make coaching mandatory. This is something that I have pushed back on in many situations. In my early work with coaching, we found great success in starting with the early adopters and then letting healthy competition and peer pressure take it from there with physicians, in particular. As a general rule, I have avoided working with organizations who wanted to mandate coaching for all and insisted on starting with the low performers. Over time, I have made a few exceptions to this, and that's been when the push for the mandate has been entirely staff driven and leadership supported. I'll share two examples, both where the idea to mandate came directly from frontline nurses. In one hospital system, we were offering care team coaching as a supportive strategy to follow some service culture training that team members had participated in. The focus was mostly with nurses, nursing assistants, health unit coordinators, or administrative support people who sat at the nursing desk and answered calls from the call light system. This hospital system was unionized, so our first stop before rolling this out was at the central unit partnership council (made up of unit council members from each service line). We shared about the opportunity and that it was entirely optional, confidential between the coach and participant, and from a positive/strengths-based approach. We then started to visit each unit partnership council and share the same information. In one mother-baby unit council, they said that they knew it was confidential between coach and participant but wondered how many would need to participate to get a cohort roll-up of their unit's particular strengths, inconsistencies, and opportunities. Given the reporting tool that we created, I am able to aggregate that data on a cohort level and agreed to do so if they had at least 10–12 sign up. Sure enough, they had about 18 nurses elect to participate!

When we went to the med-surg area of one of the hospitals in this system, they too wanted to have enough participation to aggregate their feedback. This was a large unit, and once we had coached about 30 staff, we came back to that unit partnership council and shared the results. The union members said, "This is awesome, why wouldn't we offer this to everyone? This is so supportive and affirming and educational at the same time. Let's require this for everyone who works on this unit." Thus, the mandate was born. (Figure 10.4 shows the trajectory of this med surg unit's performance.)

Spectrum of Strategies

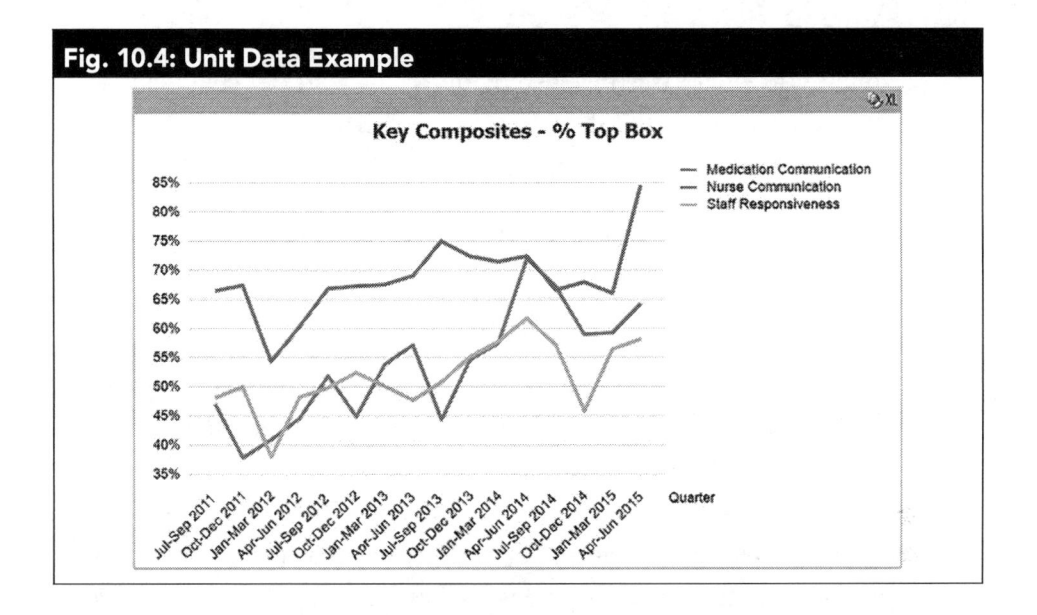

Fig. 10.4: Unit Data Example

Key Composites - % Top Box
— Medication Communication
— Nurse Communication
— Staff Responsiveness

In another organization, we were working with the trauma team of the ED. We'd started by doing some patient-level observations and mapped the care team interactions from patients' eyes. After sharing that back with the staff at various meetings, we were asked to offer coaching, optionally, to anyone who wanted to participate. We'd show up at their daily shift huddles before they went out on the floor, and the charge nurse would mention that we were there to shadow with anyone who wanted us to do so. Amazingly, more than 50 people signed up over a two-month period. Their comments about their experience help speak to the value in it for them:

- "I appreciate how the coach helps me to build on my strengths with subtle but significant changes, rather than trying an entirely new approach or rhythm."

- "The feedback was super-helpful—both encouraging in knowing what I am doing right (and that it is being noticed!) and the suggestions were specific and things that I can easily add to my everyday care."

Chapter 10

- "The coach was very unobtrusive and always showed respect and interest in what I was involved in at the moment. Her comments were very encouraging, and the input was prefaced with comments that made it easy to hear what she had to say."

- "I was able to have outside perspective on my interactions and to identify areas of improvement."

A year later when working with an interdisciplinary team of nurses, techs, physicians, and social workers in that same department, we were discussing a training program that was soon to roll out and was being made mandatory. One of the nurses spoke up and shocked me. She said, "Training is one thing, but I think the real power is in the coaching. Why wouldn't we make it mandatory that everyone have an opportunity to participate in the coaching?" And that's what they did. At the workshop the staff attended, we asked everyone to write a note to themselves entitled "My One Thing." We had them write down something they wanted to start or stop doing as a result of what they'd learned in the training session. They put it in an envelope, sealed it, and addressed it to their home address. Then, we sent the envelopes back to them about a week or so after the workshop. Each person attended the workshop, and then after that became eligible to have someone shadow and coach with them, reinforcing what they'd learned in the training session. My team coached many of them, but then we trained 10 coaches from within the department to be coaches as well.

One day, my colleague Nicole was coaching with a nurse in the department and told this person what a great job the nurse did with thanking people—patients and staff. Before Nicole could finish what she was saying, this person got a huge smile on her face and was just beaming. Nicole asked why she was smiling and the nurse said, "That was 'My One Thing' from the workshop! I wrote it on my little card, got it at home, and have been thinking about it ever since. Now you saw me in action, and it's awesome to hear that I'm actually doing it consistently!"

Spectrum of Strategies

Fig. 10.5: My One Thing Card

My one thing...

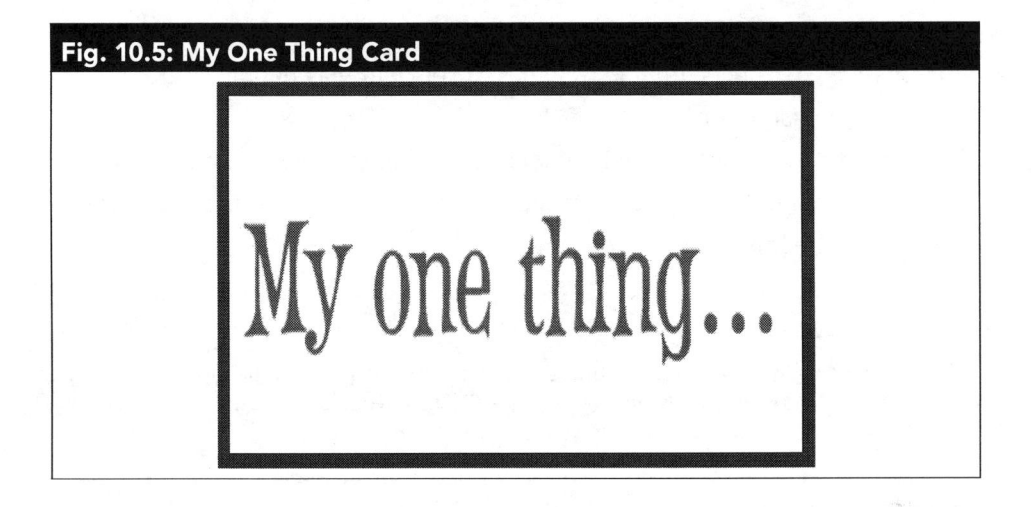

This was the best experience that I have ever been a part of where something was mandated, and yet accepted and powerful. It's not that there weren't a few staff and providers who objected, but by and large the whole department participated in the coaching and benefitted from it. The interdisciplinary team together with the department leadership just made it be the next step in the educational process; first you go to the training session, then you have an opportunity to be coached. Their scores show that the outcomes were reached (see Figure 10.6).

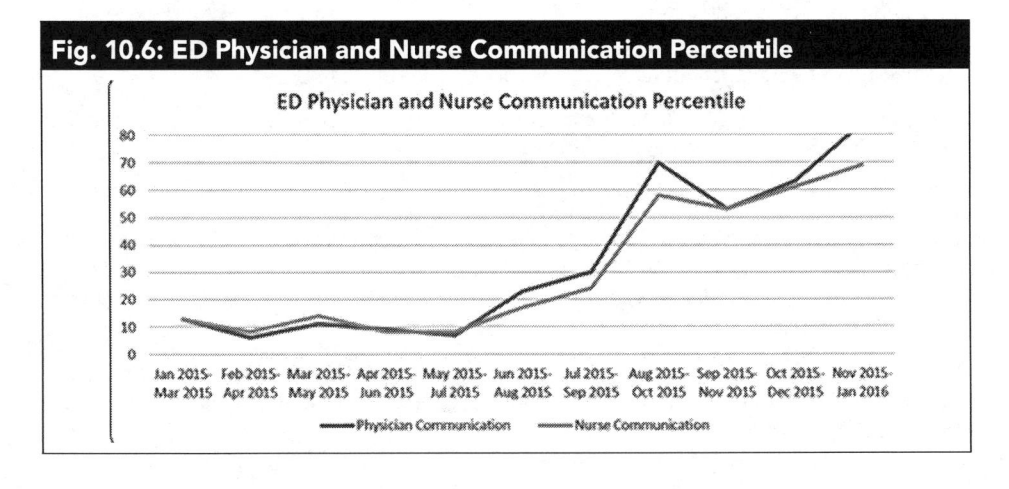

Fig. 10.6: ED Physician and Nurse Communication Percentile

ED Physician and Nurse Communication Percentile

— Physician Communication   — Nurse Communication

We've covered a variety of strategies to include in your improvement efforts. A comprehensive spectrum of strategies to consider was detailed, and we explored some additional creative ideas as well. While there still is no silver bullet in this work, we described the closest thing to it with care team coaching. Next, we'll talk about some of the potential barriers that may be encountered along the improvement journey.

References

Aligning Forces for Quality. (2012). Improving patient experience in the inpatient setting: A case study of three hospitals. Retrieved June 27, 2016, from *http://forces4quality.org/af4q/download-document/5084/Resource-Improving_Final.pdf*

Bagnasco, A., Pagnucci, N., Tolotti, A., Rosa, F., Torre, G., and Sasso, L. (2014). The role of simulation in developing communication and gestural skills in medical students. [Abstract]. *BMC Med Educ. 14: 106.* doi: 10.1186/1472-6920-14-106.

Gaba, D. (2004). The future of simulation in healthcare. *Quality and Safety in Health Care*, 13(Suppl1):i2–10.soi: 10.1136/qshc.2004009878.

Gawande, A. (2011). Personal best—Top athletes and singers have coaches. Should you? *The New Yorker.* Retrieved June 27, 2016, from *www.newyorker.com/magazine/2011/10/03/personal-best*

Okuda, Y., Bryson, E. O., DeMaria S. J., Jacobson, L., Quinones, J., Shen, B., & Levine, A. (2009). The utility of simulation in medical education: What is the evidence? [Abstract]. *Mt Sinai J Med., 76(4):* 330–43. doi: 10.1002/msj.20127.

Pascale, R., Sternin, J., and Sternin, M. (2010). *The power of Positive Deviance: How unlikely innovators solve the world's toughest problems.* Boston, MA: Harvard Business Press.

Positive Deviance Initiative (2016). Retrieved June 27, 2016, from *www.positivedeviance.org/*

Rath, T. (2007). *Strengths Finder 2.0.* New York, NY: Gallup Press.

Rath, T., and Conchie, B. (2009). *Strengths-based leadership: Great leaders, teams, and why people follow.* New York, NY: Gallup Press.

Rosen, K. (2008). The history of medical simulation. *Journal of Critical Care*, 23:157–166.

Uken, C. (2011). Billings Clinic called "pioneer" for its approach to reducing MRSA rates. *Billings Gazette.* Retrieved June 27, 2016, from *http://billingsgazette.com/news/local/billings-clinic-called-pioneer-for-its-approach-to-reducing-mrsa/article_23c5ba29-2ca4-5b68-acb9-4c71210623a4.html*

Weller, J. M., Nestel, D., Marshall, S. D., Brooks, P. M., and Conn, J. J. (2012). Simulation in clinical teaching and learning. [Abstract]. *The Medical Journal of Australia.* 196(9): 594. Doi: 10.5694/mja10.11474.

Chapter 11
Traversing the Trajectory— The Journey to Improvement

Collaboration isn't easy, and helping to keep staff and physicians engaged on the improvement journey takes a lot of effort. I think it's important to also discuss traversing a common trajectory I like to call the "Puke or Shoot Continuum." I've experienced this many times over with both physicians and care team members.

No one likes to be sick, and let's face it—puking is the worst. Second to that, I guess, is getting puked on. If you have had kids or have been around them, especially if one of them gets carsick easily, then you know what I mean.

After speaking to many groups about communication and patient experience —especially when I had the distinct privilege of being the first or one of the first people to speak to a group of doctors about CMS; public transparency of these data; what the HCAHPS, CG CAHPS, or ED CAHPS surveys are; the questions, the wording, the scoring methodology, etc.—I began to notice a pattern. One of two things would happen: They'd either shoot the messenger or puke on the data. I saw how groups had to go through various stages of the acceptance process (very thankful for my social work roots here). It takes some time and discussion to help groups get over their frustrations and doubts to the point where they are ready to make changes and hear how they could improve. Sometimes a group can move through this process in one meeting or conversation. Sometimes it takes a series of conversations over time.

Here are some points on the Puke or Shoot Continuum.

- **Don't shoot!** In this stage, people tend to either shoot the messenger or puke on the data. And let's be honest, sometimes it's both of these in the same conversation! This is where a lot of the frustrations often surface about CMS, public transparency, the survey tools, etc. The most common issues or concerns I hear are things such as:

    - "Why does only 'Always' count? Everyone can have a bad day once in a while. No one is perfect."

    - "The response rates are so low. We see 30,000 patients a year and you want me to believe a sample of 30–90 responses? That's not in any way reflective of our population!"

    - "This survey is reflective of more than my piece of the journey. They may be thinking of things that occurred before they got to me. I can't play catch-up if things have already gone wrong."

If you find yourself in a place where these concerns are coming at you, a natural reaction is to be defensive. Rather than try to defend, I try to use humor. I'll say something like, "Hey, I hear you. Believe me, I have my list for CMS, but they didn't ask me when they were putting this all together." It's important to acknowledge this skepticism as valid and healthy and even name it as part of this journey. Whatever you can do to invite this and let them get it out will help. It's not a good idea to rush a group through this stage or to try to dismiss their concerns and move on.

Using the improv skill of "Yes, and" is helpful in this phase. After letting them be heard and getting it all out, it's a good idea to try to use some humor and also help hold them in some of the reality of the situation. If someone says, "This is ridiculous. How can I be held accountable for these things that are influenced by so many other people in this patient's journey?" then you could respond with, "Yes, that feels unfair. And it's also true of so many of our other established quality metrics, right? Like readmissions, look at how many people play a role in that."

Try your best to calmly present the rationale behind the surveys and the payment structure. This is where the video I referenced earlier is a helpful way to explain this to a group: *What the Heck Is Value-Based Purchasing?* (Visit *www.youtube.com/watch?v=dF8SGblP7-c* .)

- **"My patients are different!"** This is where some will make the case for exemptions, declaring that their patients are sicker, more negative, or should be otherwise excluded from the CMS and public reporting. I had one neurologist in a Midwest town look me straight in the eyes and declare that his patients in his practice were in more pain than any other patients of a neurology practice anywhere else in the country! I find that by letting folks be heard with their concerns and then talking about the national movement and transparency of the data to compare patients from all regions can help.

- **"Show me my data!"** This is when physicians or nurses want to see how they individually do—not as a group, a hospital, a clinic, a unit, or a department. Although HCAHPS asks questions about doctors or nurses, groups are able to achieve huge success with transparency of data through customized individual-level reports or use of an EDW to get at individual physician-level data. I've also worked with EDs that were able to get some of their experience-related postdischarge call information stratified by nurses and providers.

- **"Tell me what the patients say!"** I love it when a group gets to this point because they are coming around and want to know what their patients are saying. This is where the value of talking to patients about the specifics of communication—through focus groups or Patient & Family Advisory Councils—can project that patient voice which so readily resonates with physicians and frontline staff.

- **"Fine, just tell me what to do."** This is my favorite point: when a group is ready to hear how they may make an impact and are open to the various strategies that can help improve their communication with patients. At this point, it is crucial to be ready with the two to three improvement strategies you'd suggest that the group employ to help improve their communication.

Please hear me on this: I love working with physicians and other care team members! I don't say any of this to disparage or stereotype. I just am calling out a pattern that I have seen time and again. As I work with groups all over the country, when I describe this Puke or Shoot Continuum, it resonates. I find that this gives those of us working in this space a language for our common experiences. One of my favorite CNOs called me and said, "I think we got through the 'Don't shoot' phase, but now we're stuck on the 'Show me my data' phase!" Together we talked about some tips for how to help her med exec group get unstuck as we worked out a model for attribution of the HCAHPS data at the physician level. Once they were able to move on with their own data, they were able to start to make some meaningful improvements and progress on this path of performance.

You're on the Journey, Now What?

What do you do if you find yourself on the Puke or Shoot Continuum? Below are some tips on how to get started, and help groups move through this process and on to improvement in communication.

1. **Don't get stuck in analysis paralysis.**

   When it comes to data and improvement strategies, don't let *great* get in the way of *good,* and just get started! At the same time, pause long enough to ask the patients first what they'd like to see. Examine what they are already telling you through their comments, complaints, and conversations. Also, be mindful of what else they can readily tell you through the use of Patient and Family Advisory Councils and focus groups.

2. **Don't chase your tail.**

   In other words, don't focus on the left side of the bell-shaped curve—that is, the "Never" responses to the questions. Without fail, when groups look at their survey responses, someone will say, "Can't we just find out whose patients said, 'Never'? Let's just deal with those physicians caring for them and we'll be all set!"

   Well, the answer is no. CAHPS surveys only report the top-box percentages. Instead of trying to eliminate the "Nevers," focus on moving the "Usually" responses to "Always." To do this means improving consistency and also exceeding patient expectations. All we're trying to do is move the "Usuallys" to "Always" and ensure some healthy competition. From strictly a numbers or CAHPS perspective, all you need to do is move the bell-shaped curve to the right. Focusing on the outliers or the "Nevers" will not, in and of itself, get you substantial numerical success.

3. **Focus on the few and the furious.**

   Be methodical, logical, and reasonable when it comes to goals for improvement. If you implement five things at once, how do you know what works and what does not? When you can furiously focus on a few specific goals and strategies, your messages will be clearer to the physicians and team, and you'll be more likely to recognize early success and create strong momentum.

Realize that this work will take time. There may be pilots that don't work or ideas that don't yield what you hope. If you can stay the course, though, it is genuinely possible to achieve transformational success.

4. **Find your partners in crime.**

   It takes a village to realize success in this work. Building a core team of physicians and staff who care about this as much as you do is essential to achieving and sustaining results.

5. **Get the word out!**

   Communication is essential, and consistency is vital to getting your message out. Get on the agenda at staff meetings and provider meetings, use newsletters and blogs, and make it part of ongoing conversations. And once you start, don't stop!

6. **Improvement won't just happen.**

   The reality is that if it were easy, it would already be done. Organizations that have achieved success have chosen to be committed and have made it a priority to make a difference. The good news is that the reward is well worth it—certainly for the team, but, ultimately, for the patients.

How does this all tie back to traversing the Puke or Shoot Continuum? These five tips and the spectrum of strategies that we've covered in this book can be of assistance.

Traversing the Trajectory—The Journey to Improvement

Traversing the Trajectory	Path to Performance
"Don't shoot!"	• It takes a village! • This is where I see those partners in crime—the core team of physicians, leaders, and frontline staff who care about this as much as you do who can help support and reinforce the improvement efforts. I'm struck by how often the pushback occurs outside of the formal meeting, on the unit, in the pod, in the lounge—and that's where it's so important to have allies to help calmly hear and appropriately challenge their peers.
"My patients are different!"	• This is where being comfortable enough with the compulsories to freely discuss public transparency is important. • Reinforcing that this applies to nearly every hospital everywhere is helpful.
"Show me my data!"	• Here is where data shines ... being ready with appropriate data quality and visualization to help get to the most meaningful level of granularity that your data can support (physician, group, unit, etc.).
"Tell me what my patients say!"	• It is essential that you project the patient voices. • Draw upon their comments, councils, complaints, and any sources of their thoughts and wishes.
"Fine, just tell me what to do!"	• Be ready with the improvement strategies for what you want them to do! • Coaching, training, care boards, sitting down—choose the options that fit with your organization's chosen path and be ready to help them engage!

I was at a patient experience conference recently and one of the physicians from an organization that we'd been working with decided to attend. He'd spent a few days at the conference really just taking it all in. He was a self-admitted skeptic, so I was impressed that he had even chosen to attend in the first place! As we walked down the street to the evening event, he said, "I'm still not sure I'm convinced ..." and he went on to talk about his beef with CMS, the data, etc. As we chatted, I was struck by the dichotomy between his concerns and his success. As a leader within his group, he'd helped to create so much of the great work that led to that organization's improvement. And

Chapter 11

yet, he himself still had his own frustrations and concerns with the system. This conversation reinforced again to me how much this is an ongoing journey of continuing connection and collaboration.

The next two chapters highlight some of the stories from organizations who have achieved some success while traversing this trajectory. I know, because I've been with both of them on this journey over the years. It hasn't been an easy road, and we've all learned some key lessons along the way. They graciously have shared the details of the multiple efforts they used to help realize their goals.

Chapter 12
Case Study: Allina Health

by Steve Bergeson, Tracy Laibson, and Janet Wied

Organizational Background

Allina Health is a nonprofit health system consisting of clinics, hospitals, and other health services, providing care throughout Minnesota and western Wisconsin. Allina Health employs over 27,000, and in 2015 had 4.3 million clinic visits, 1.4 million hospital outpatient visits, and just over 109,000 inpatient admissions. Allina Health cares for patients from beginning to end-of-life through its 90+ clinics, 13 hospitals, 15 pharmacies, specialty care centers, and specialty medical services that provide home care, senior transitions, hospice care, home oxygen and medical equipment, and emergency medical transportation services.

Historical Context

As an organization, Allina's patient experience focus started around data. In the early to mid-2000s, the formal work was around its patient satisfaction surveying at the system office. Patient satisfaction data was measured, and was part of the corporate scorecards, so it was seen as important. However, the ability to segment data was limited, and it was difficult to get the results to the end users. System steering teams for patient satisfaction (eventually termed "patient experience") were focused on data and measurement. Performance improvement occurred in pockets throughout the hospitals and clinics. There was no formal coordination between the hospitals or business units (regions/clinics), so work was independent and siloed.

Prior to the requirements of HCAHPS for the hospitals and CG CAHPS for the clinics, Allina used homegrown, locally administered surveys. The results seemed to be positive, but Allina had no external benchmarks for comparison. In the ambulatory and hospital divisions, quality measures (clinical core measures and other metrics) were the initial focus for improvement efforts. Patient experience came later. Once the hospitals and clinics moved to standardized, benchmarked, required survey tools, they found their patients rated them about average for patient experience, in contrast to the top quartile for quality. This led to more structured support for performance improvement.

Early attempts at formal mandates for patient experience standardization across hospitals (i.e., hourly rounding) were not successful due to decentralized leadership coupled with the union environment.

In 2009, a system patient experience director role was created and site leads (individuals with other formal roles serving as the informal patient experience point of contact) at each hospital were identified. In 2010, a director of patient experience in the ambulatory division was established. Both patient experience directors created teams to support the work across the system and within their key areas of focus. They focused on support for the sites/local units. Physician leadership for patient experience has been a component on the ambulatory side dating back to early 2000s. Physician champions emerged in 2010 and were key to the inpatient work and improvement as well.

Executive leadership for this work has changed often, leading to vacillations between system office– and business unit–directed approaches to improvement.

Current and Recent Activity

Given this backdrop, Allina has achieved some remarkable success and gained traction through a multitude of efforts over the past seven years. Some supporting activities that have contributed to their overall success in patient experience include:

- Patient experience steering committees have developed and taken various forms and structures over the years.
- Care boards were standardized across all of the hospitals.
- Shadow coaching was provided for hospitalists, specialists, and physicians in the clinics.
- Targeted improvements and goals were set for key domains and composites. Within the ambulatory division, focus was paid to the domains of "access to care" and provider communication, especially the question of whether or not the "provider knew my medical history." Within the hospital division, specific focused work in physician communication, pain management, environmental cleanliness, and nursing communication led to success in each of those composites.
- Nurse leaders rounding on "every patient, every stay" was adopted in the inpatient areas.
- Standard greeting and closing scripts for staff talking to patients on the phone were implemented across the clinics.
- Uniforms were standardized for staff across the hospitals.
- Development of "Our Promise" coincided with the rebranding to Allina Health (see Figure 12.1). This was used in recruitment and to translate the mission and vision for the organization into tangible statements to each other and to patients.

Fig. 12.1: Allina Promise

Our promise

We are all here to help you on your path to better health.
Every one of us.
Here to care, to guide, to motivate, to comfort, to inspire.

The work we do is profound and distinguishes us.
But it's the small things we do every day that will define us.

We believe you are an integral part of the care team.
We are here in service to you, from beginning to end.
Dedicated to enriching your experience with us —
body, mind and spirit.
Whenever, wherever we meet.

On your path with us, we will give you options.
We will respect your time.
We will use plain language.
We will listen with compassion.
And speak with purpose.
We will applaud your efforts.
We will address concerns.

We will be fearless advocates and tireless partners
on your path to better health.

Allina Health

Case Study: Allina Health

- Aligned service standards, called "Our Commitment to Care," were implemented across the organization.

- "Care on the Spot," a recognition program, was developed to align recognition with the service standards. Additionally, high-performing physicians and units/sites are recognized in a variety of manners.

- Videos to demonstrate specific actions and key communication practices were created and shared with staff and physicians.

In addition, there have been several other recent key strategies. Given how each of these are integral to the current and future success, a deeper dive was warranted.

Patient and Family Partnership Program

Allina Health has had a Patient Advisory Council (PAC) program since 2009. In 2014, a project began to redesign the program to make it more robust and sustainable and include means of engaging patients in various ways. A team of Allina Health employees and patients developed the Patient and Family Partnership Program (PFPP) model in October 2014. This program is designed on the concept of "Nothing about me, without me."

At the core of the PFPP is a pool of patient and family partners (more than 100 after one year into the program, and growing) recruited through *AllinaHealth.org*, social media, and the recommendations of frontline staff. These partners serve as advisors to the work at Allina Health. To involve patients in planning and strategy across the care continuum, there are five tiers of participation: Allina-wide PFAC, Focus Groups, eAdvisors, Committee Participation, and Patient and Family Panels.

Chapter 12

Fig. 12.2: Allina Patient and Family Partnership Program

[Diagram: Patient & Family Partnership Program — Focus Groups, E-advisors, Patient & Family Advisory Council (center), Committees & Projects, Patient Panels, all supported by Patient and Family Advisors. Allina Health.]

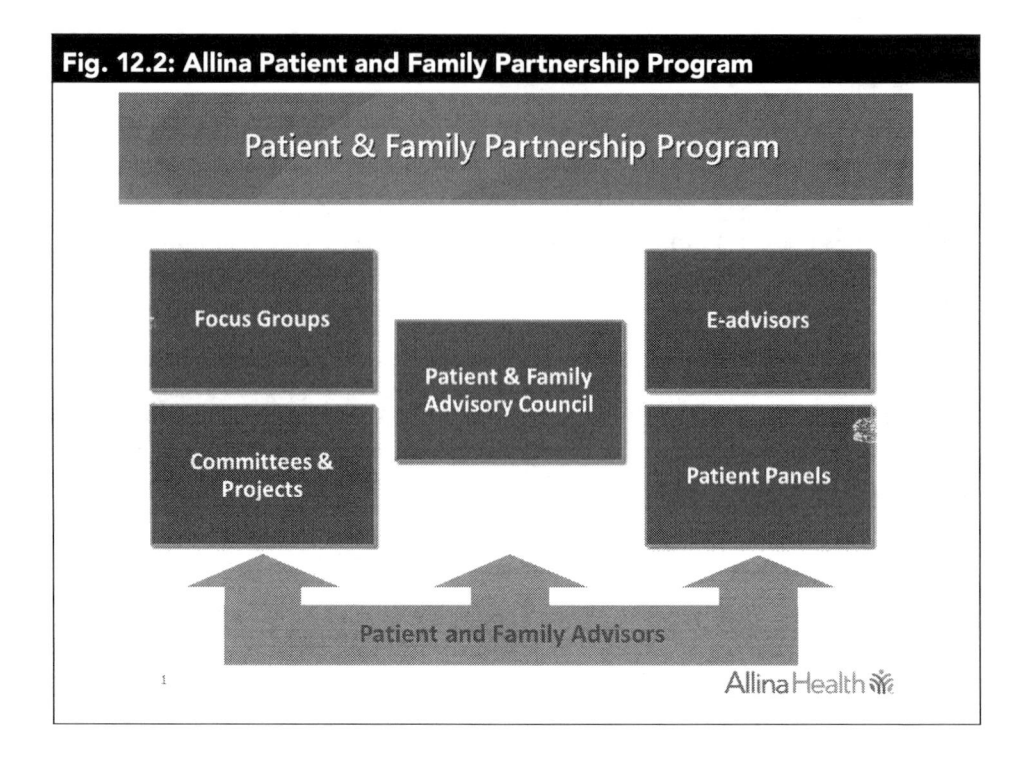

The PFPP is designed to overcome some of the challenges of Allina Health's prior PAC program structure. One key change was having stakeholders within the organization engaged in the councils and focus groups to hear the advisor insights firsthand.

Chief Medical Officer Timothy Sielaff, MD, PhD, was very clear: "Patients and families can drive our agenda better or as well as our scores can. Bring patients in and they will change the conversation … we should have them present."

Rolling out the new program included communication and education to ensure stakeholders requesting patient and family insights were oriented to the goals of the program and the guiding principles for successful engagement of the patient and family voice. Allina Health has developed a four-stage process for every patient and family advisor engagement throughout the organization:

Case Study: Allina Health

1. Readiness Assessment—Assess the needs and readiness of staff requesting patient and family advisors:

- What are we trying to learn? What are we ready to hear?
- Who are we trying to learn from? Who are the stakeholders involved?
- Where might we gather input?
- What are we currently doing to gather input?
- How do we want to gather input?
- When do we want to gain input?

2. Planning—Prepare for a successful partnership:

- Define the patient and family participant role.
- Identify and include key stakeholders.
- Recruit patients, families, and/or community members for formal screening/interview process.
- Coordinate meeting logistics.

3. Engagement—Prepare staff and advisors to work together with the following guidelines:

- Clearly define roles of stakeholders and PFPP advisors.
- Display a positive and supportive attitude toward the mission of Allina Health.
- Respect the perspectives of others by listening to differing opinions and different points of view.
- Foster a safe and supportive environment for open dialogue.
- Show concern for more than one issue or agenda.

Chapter 12

- Work in close partnership with others.
- Allow the discussion to take a different direction than anticipated.

4. Follow-up—Share and utilize input, and follow through with advisors:

- Summarize the input thoroughly and honestly.
- Share the input more broadly across the system.
- Create an action plan for using the input.
- Report back to participants and families on use of the input.
- Debrief with Allina Health Patient Experience teams.

Follow-up is key to success with this work. Patient advisors have had negative experiences with this type of work when they feel that all they are doing is talking to each other. While they don't expect everything they share to be implemented, they need to feel they are being heard. Allina Health shares written summaries of the insights from the PFPP across the organization and has patient and family advisors meet with groups to present takeaways from their council meetings and focus groups. A member of the patient experience team regularly communicates with PFPP members about the outcomes of their insights being shared and utilized within Allina Health.

Engaging patients and family members as partners in the work of a healthcare organization is essential. Allina Health has also found that creating and following clear guiding principles around that engagement process is required for success. This is an ongoing journey, as the focus on consumerism in healthcare continues to expand. Allina Health recently created a Consumer Insights Advisory Council with membership from departments across the organization, plus patient and community members, to ensure the organization continues to be proactive and intentional in the engagement of the patient, family, consumer, and community member voice in shaping the direction of the work.

"When we speak to a group at Allina Health, it is clear people are paying attention to what we say. People are taking notes, asking questions, and listening."

—Patient and family advisor

"I appreciate the commitment from our patients—giving of their time, voice, and heart. Hearing firsthand what they experienced, what is important to them, and what would be helpful is very valuable."

—Allina Health staff member

"We have to take the voice of the patient and the voice of their families into things to understand what is really most meaningful and most impactful … By continuing to work with our patient and family advisors, we can transform and enhance the care our patients receive and create an even better patient experience for the future."

—Penny Wheeler, Allina Health CEO

Data

Allina Health is a data-driven organization, and patient experience is no exception. When CMS implemented HCAHPS in 2006, Allina Health had already been surveying patients in much of the organization about their satisfaction (as it was called then) for several years. Allina Health decided to become certified as its own HCAHPS vendor since it was already administering all of its own surveys. For two years, the primary focus of the small patient experience staff was survey administration, processing, and reporting.

In 2009, the decision was made to partner with a vendor for survey administration (beginning with HCAHPS and slowly expanding to all other surveying) so that the Allina Health staff with patient experience roles (portions of two FTEs at that time) could focus on data analysis and performance improvement.

Chapter 12

In 2008, Allina Health began development of an EDW. The EDW allowed for integration of EMR data with a variety of other data sources, and reporting dashboards were built to provide users with easy access to data in the EDW. One requirement of the patient experience survey vendor was to return raw data files of the survey results to Allina Health. In 2010, those patient survey results data were built into the EDW to connect it with the EMR and other data sources, and enable extensive options for associating patient experience survey results with various patient demographic and clinical information.

A patient experience dashboard was built to allow highly customizable reporting access to the data, and patient experience results were included in many other dashboards (clinical service lines, care management, and readmissions, etc.) to support the use of patient experience survey results as a key metric aligned with all organizational initiatives. The Clinical Leadership Team approved full internal transparency of data down to the provider level in 2010. Across the system, people put effort into making that data accessible, understood, and actionable.

Patient experience collaboratives

A senior clinic leader asked a question in 2012: "Could a focused approach with a group of clinics for a defined period of time using improvement methods combined with accountability foster more rapid improvement than working with all clinics at once?" The patient experience collaboratives were the result of this question. Leadership and accountability were applied in a focused approach to improvement based on the Institute for Healthcare Improvement's Breakthrough Collaborative model.

During the six months of the collaborative, which was implemented on a regional basis, additional improvement resources were available to clinics, including process improvement, measurement, shadowing resources for individual clinicians, and resources to coach clinic leaders in improvement methods.

Case Study: Allina Health

The collaboratives were built on two activities: 1) a multidisciplinary Service Action Team (SAT) focused on clinicwide interventions to improve the patient experience, and 2) a focus on provider communication by clinicians and clinician leaders.

The SAT focused both on known interventions to improve the patient experience, which might not be consistently applied currently, as well as innovations not in current practice. Known interventions not consistently applied in Allina terms are "must-haves." Examples of known interventions not consistently applied were: the "Ten-Four" rule (at 10 feet away, you make eye contact with people, and at 4 feet away, you greet them); walking out to greet the patient, instead of calling patients from the doorway; waiting room introductions by staff with their name and role; and walking with patients between settings in the clinic with warm handoffs to the next person. Examples of innovations were: a different-colored routing slip for patients new to the practice; scripts to accompany the new routing slips; methods to apprise patients of waiting times (e.g., tracking boards, yellow and red cards, checking in every 10–15 minutes, and apprising of waits); and offering coffee and water for waiting patients. Innovations in early collaboratives that were successful often became must-haves in subsequent collaboratives.

Provider communication was addressed through a Clinician Improvement Plan (CLIP) for clinicians with provider communication scores below the 50th national percentile. The process was nondisciplinary and encouraged clinicians to choose one specific action to work on over a defined period of time, with assessments built in to determine if the action was being consistently applied. One-on-one follow-up meetings with clinician leaders were held at 30, 60, and 90 days to ascertain if the actions were being implemented, and to encourage and guide clinicians as they chose additional actions. Examples of actions clinicians implemented successfully were knocking and pausing before entering an exam room, demonstrating to the patient they knew the medical history, and making personal connections during the visit. Practicing teach back was found to be complex and not a starting place for most clinicians. Clinicians on CLIPs had the option of being shadowed by a nonclinician to assess their clinic interactions through a layperson's eyes. One surprise during the CLIP process was the discomfort that clinician leaders—who were experienced at coaching on clinician issues like diabetes care—felt with coaching their colleagues to improve nonclinical aspects of care like the patient experience.

Significant time was spent developing patient experience skills during the collaborative and timelines for the follow-up meetings with clinicians. Process metrics were the mainstay of measurement, and many of these were based on observation or self-assessment. The challenge for teams was to measure enough to ensure a change was making a difference without burdensome measurement. Normal work continued at each clinic, so many were tired at the end of each collaborative. Fun and celebration were parts of each collaborative, with awards done in creative and funny ways to thank and celebrate teams for their improvement.

The first collaborative with one region (nine clinics) was deemed successful enough to spread to two regions at a time (six to nine clinics each), and this method was maintained through the two years of the collaborative so that every clinic in the division across all regions had the opportunity to experience the collaborative. Clinicwide initiatives continued during the collaboratives, such as videos on first impressions and "Narrating the Visit," as well as a focus on provider communication and ensuring patient comments were reviewed and acted upon.

Patient experience scores improved during each collaborative, and over the course of the two years, improved from the 35th national percentile for "Willingness to Recommend" to close to the 70th national percentile. Provider communication improved more rapidly for the clinicians involved in the CLIP process than for those who were not. As a result of the shadowing experience available to clinicians on CLIPs, all new clinicians are now being shadowed in their first three to four months of employment to help their adjustment to the clinic. Not every clinic and not every clinician improved, and some of the ongoing work is to determine ways to help those below goal improve and develop additional approaches.

Now that the collaboratives have ended, the idea of taking focused approaches to improvements is still incorporated. The key initiatives identified during the collaboratives, such as walking with the patients to the room, narrating the visit, and distinctive routing slips for new patients, are still standard across the division.

Bedside Shift Handover

In 2014, Allina Health made the decision to implement bedside shift handover as a standard inpatient practice at all the hospitals. There is no chief nursing officer across the system, so the patient experience department works with the collaborative Nurse Executive Council (NEC)—a committee of the senior nursing director or vice president at each hospital—on nursing-related patient experience initiatives. That group became the executive sponsors of bedside shift handover.

As a multihospital system without centralized hospital leadership (Allina Health has now developed a regional structure with the triad of region leaders sharing hospital divisionwide leadership), a key to any patient experience initiative being implemented across all hospitals is determining what will be standardized and what will be up to local design. Individual hospitals are the implementation owners, with the hospital division patient experience team providing subject matter expertise, advice, tools, and resources, and the NEC maintaining decision-making authority and accountability. This was the case for the bedside shift handover work.

Chapter 12

The first step was to determine the must-haves for an Allina Health bedside shift handover experience. Patient experience staff reviewed best practice and approaches from other healthcare organizations, and the NEC agreed to five components that must be part of every handover:

1. Introduction of the oncoming nurse

2. Care board update

3. Discussion of patients' pain and comfort

4. Review of goals and plan of care

5. Patient participation

Hospitals were free to include other components they chose to require locally. After several months of implementation, a sixth component—safety checks—was added as a requirement of all hospitals because one hospital had been using it and found it extremely valuable. The balance between standardization and local approaches allows for learning from practices at individual hospitals while continuing to evolve a standardized approach.

The nurse executives assessed that their hospitals and units were at various stages of readiness to implement bedside shift handover. The decision was made to allow a full year for implementation—hospitals could phase the rollout as they deemed appropriate, with the expectation that all hospitals have full handover with required components in place on all inpatient units by year end. Patient experience is on the NEC agenda monthly, and the group used this time to discuss successes and challenges throughout the implementation process.

A member of the hospital division patient experience team developed a bedside shift handover toolkit to serve as an implementation and, eventually, hardwiring/sustainability resource for the hospitals. This toolkit includes information on what bedside shift handover is, the goals of using it, why it is important to patients/families and to nurses (including comments from both groups), how it connects to Allina Health's service standards, and an overview of the must-have components. The toolkit also provides information on how to develop an implementation team, details to consider when developing the bedside shift handover process and workflow, and recommendations for training and ongoing accountability. A few months into the implementation process, Allina Health added a detailed list of barriers to completing bedside shift handover (based on what we were hearing from nurses) and suggested responses and ways to address those barriers.

Most hospitals engaged members of their unit councils to develop the implementation plan, training process, etc. Performance improvement or patient experience team members were involved to help operationalize and facilitate this.

Each quarter, Allina Health's patient care managers from across hospitals come together for a half-day meeting. One of these meetings was dedicated to bedside shift handover during the implementation period. The goal was to make a strong connection between bedside shift handover and the Allina Health service standards. The session included a presentation from a successful early adopter unit, demonstrations of doing bedside shift handover right and wrong, and practice and role-playing by the attendees.

Once all hospitals had put the bedside shift handover requirement in place, the patient experience team developed a process for assessing frequency and quality of occurrence. To avoid the negative associations with an audit, this was rolled out as a bedside shift handover spot-check process. For one 24-hour period, every off-going nurse was asked how many patients he or she had been assigned and how many he or she had completed bedside shift handover for. Each nurse was also asked to comment on successes and barriers. This quantitative data was helpful for the nurse executives at each hospital to discuss opportunities and strengths and plan for improvement. The qualitative data about successes and barriers was incredibly valuable in

Chapter 12

identifying the key challenges left to address (e.g., clarifying the process for sleeping patients), and provided some stories of safety catches that occurred during handover and other reasons many nurses were finding the process valuable. These were incorporated into the toolkit.

Once all hospitals had completed implementing the expectation of bedside shift handover with the six must-haves, NEC discussed the next steps in getting to consistent, quality use of bedside shift handover. Three key projects were identified:

1. Make the bedside shift handover spot-check a quarterly process for ongoing measurement and accountability. Some hospitals opted to do the spot-check more frequently, but only collect and report to the system quarterly.

2. Develop a formal competency assessment with learning and development. This has not been made a requirement, but is available for those who want to use it. One hospital, which has seen significant improvement in their HCAHPS communication with nurses and overall rating, has opted to require the competency assessment for all inpatient nurses. This has allowed them to assume a baseline knowledge and then hold nurses accountable for consistent use of bedside shift handover. Nurses also do peer-to-peer audits and observations of the practice.

3. Add bedside shift handover to the Allina-wide hospital nurse orientation. Many new nurses come in having learned about bedside shift handover as a standard practice. There are even stories of nurses opting not to work at hospitals that do not require the practice. Once the requirement was implemented across hospitals, it could be added to standardized orientation for all new nurses.

Allina Health's EDs have also started implementing bedside shift handover in pockets. The patient experience team created a toolkit specific to the process in the ED setting. There is not a plan to make this a system standard at this time, but those who have implemented the process find it valuable.

Implementing bedside shift handover as a standard practice across inpatient units has resulted in a consistent increase in patients' rating of nursing communication on HCAHPS surveys. Similar increases occurred in ratings of pain management and staff responsiveness, which are also impacted by the bedside shift handover practice. Opportunity remains around consistency and some individuals who still resist this change in practice. Nurse and hospital leaders are encouraged to be present, and to round on units during change of shift to encourage bedside shift handover and recognize those who are using the practice. Ongoing spot-checks show continued improvement in consistency overall.

From Allina Health patients

- "I can't emphasize enough the importance of the bedside handoff. It made me feel safe, like I was part of my plan of care, and that I could correct any information that wasn't accurate."

- "Bedside handoff was impressive, I loved not having to tell my story over again to the next nurse and felt very involved."

- "I really liked during the change of shift how both nurses would be in the room with me and pass on all the info to the next nurse on duty. I can't say enough about them. Thank you."

- "I missed the handoff when it wasn't done."

From Allina Health nurses

- "I get my eyes on the patients and literally can see if things look okay."

Chapter 12

- "It gives me the opportunity to ask questions I might not otherwise have thought to ask because I am seeing the patient."

- "Patients contribute good information."

- "Patients are using call lights less."

- "Helps me get out on time."

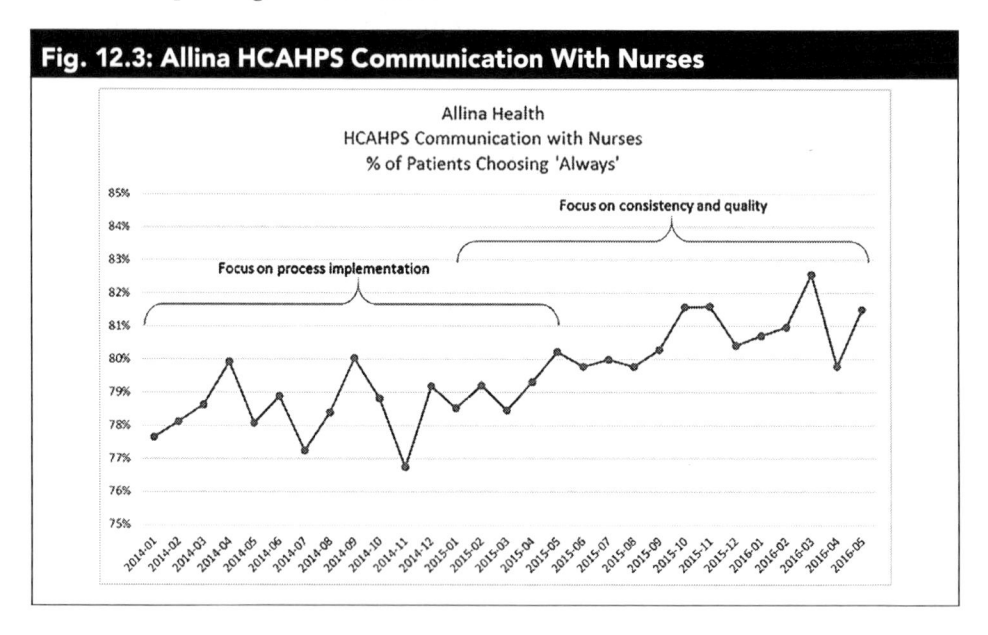

Fig. 12.3: Allina HCAHPS Communication With Nurses

Results

As a result of the collective work across the various initiatives detailed in this chapter, Allina Health has seen significant improvement in all of the HCAHPS and CG CAHPS composites across their inpatient and outpatient areas. Highlighted here are two of the overall metrics of their success.

Case Study: Allina Health

Fig. 12.4: Allina HCAHPS Overall Rating

Fig. 12.5: Allina Willingness to Recommend Control Chart

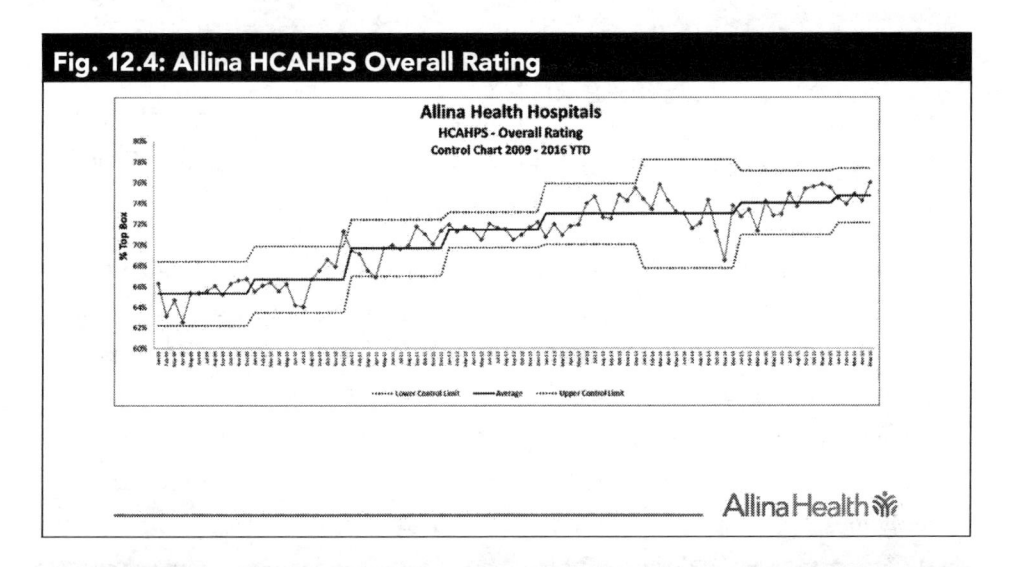

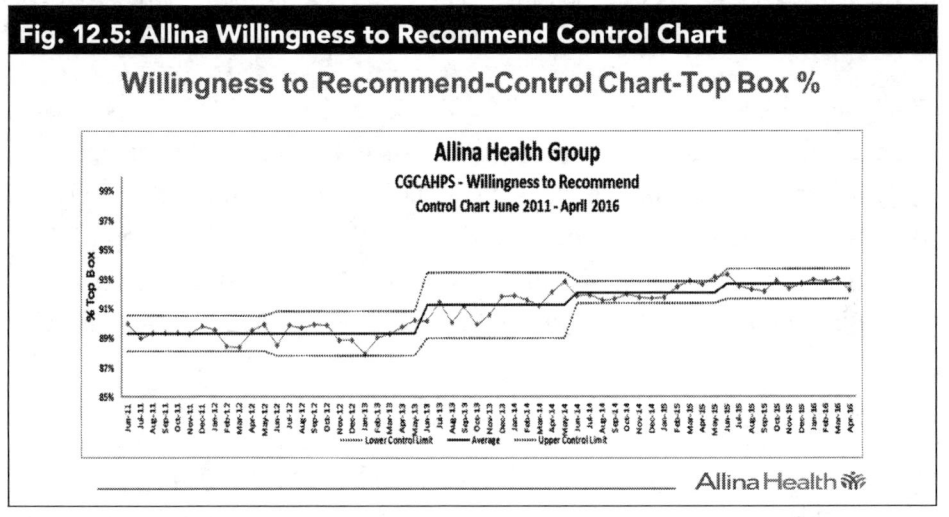

Lessons Learned

Despite these successes, the Allina team has identified several key lessons learned along the way.

Chapter 12

Leadership approach

All of the greatest ideas in the world from staff and management will not get much traction if senior leaders are not on board and setting the tone. This has been true in the patient experience journey at Allina.

Allina Health has always had leadership that believed a focus on patient experience was a good idea (hard to argue against it!), but in 2012 it began to receive more attention. Allina's CEO at that time took a strong stance on the importance of patient experience and the need for it to be top of mind. He challenged the organization not only to be in the top quartile in performance by 2015—he also advocated for the 90th percentile in overall achievement. In weekly messages, he wrote about it often. One particular message was especially important as he described his reasons for considering patient experience so important for us to focus on at Allina Health.

First, he explained, it is an issue of practicality—financial health depends on it as organizations are rewarded (or penalized) based on patient experience performance. Second, patient experience is an important part of overall quality. One completes the other. Third and most important, this approach is required to pass the "What would I want for my Mom?" test. Messages like this from senior leaders were critical in getting everyone on the same page.

Accountability

Just as senior leadership needs to set the tone, everyone needs to be held accountable to execute on plans and implement agreed-upon tactics. This was an area in the health group where a change was in order.

Allina's patient experience leaders worked hard to develop tactics and plans, refined reporting to make it meaningful, and communicated to the sites what was expected, and assumed it was happening. It was only when a new health group senior leader asked the patient experience staff to find out if it was really happening that it was uncovered that in many cases it was not.

Regional leaders needed to be clear with site leaders and staff that this was not optional work. Deadlines were expected to be met, plans were expected to be turned in, and when not, it was escalated up to their leader(s) to investigate and course correct. This was difficult at first and not always well received. It was not about people not wanting to do the right thing—many times, it was all the other things that got in the way. Sometimes, it was the need to have a crucial conversation with a clinician or staff member that they felt unprepared for. Part of the role of the patient experience team was to assist in removing those barriers so the work could be done. You cannot assume that what you want to happen, does happen. You need to use continuous improvement methodology to check back and study what is happening (or not), course correct if necessary, and move forward. Accountability is very similar to the PDSA cycle. They work together to bring improvement over time.

Centralization

In many organizations, there is a chief experience officer and a central Office of Patient Experience. Allina continues to look for the right structure and resourcing to support their informal alignment. Despite not having a formal, central structure, the divisions of the organization work collaboratively. For example, Allina Health Group patient experience team manages the ongoing physician shadow coaching across the system and the hospital division patient experience team manages the PFPP across the system.

Standardization vs. innovation

This is an ongoing debate at Allina. How many tactics and initiatives should be standard across all hospitals or clinics, and how much should be left to the individual unit or site? And does it really matter? The patient experience leaders think it does, although some other leaders feel differently. It is a balancing act and Allina Health continues working to find the right balance.

In working with patient and family advisors, they say they expect certain parts of their experience to be standard across Allina Health, or at a minimum across all clinics or all hospitals. It is comforting to them to know what to expect as they interact with the system. Those are the basics, or foundational things, that we know make a difference. They are the simple things (or should be simple), such as knocking before entering a room, introducing yourself if patients or families are new to you, narrating what you are doing, conducting bedside shift handover with nursing, and thanking them for allowing you to care for them, to name a few. These need to be hardwired, consistent, and reliable before work on those exciting, extra things that will wow patients. While there is little pushback that these are the right things to do, there are differences of opinion as to whether it matters how they get implemented. The clinics have had the most success by implementing in a standard fashion, while the hospitals have taken the approach to implementation in a manner that works for each hospital or department. Both are showing improvement on a year-over-year basis, so the debate continues.

Where Is Allina Health Headed?

Like most large healthcare organizations today, Allina Health is faced with many changes and the challenges they bring moving from:

- A fee-for-service to a value-based payment world
- Caring only for those who enter our doors to taking responsibility for all in the communities we serve
- A focus on healing to a commitment to well-being
- Looking at patient interactions as transactions to relationships based on whole-person care

Allina Health is entering into an ever-increasing digital world, causing it to look at new and different ways to provide care.

Physician and staff burnout is increasing in healthcare. Consequently, Allina Health is working on tools and tactics to assist leaders and caregivers to be more resilient in the face of all this change. Providing an excellent patient experience can make us more resilient. Physicians who have strong positive relationships with their patients are also more satisfied in the work they are doing, which can decrease the feelings of burnout.

Work continues to establish and reinforce a strong, vibrant, and positive culture across the organization that reflects what we want to bring to our communities. Allina Health increasingly looks to patients, families, and communities, as well as employees, to engage in this work. Ultimately, the focus is on long-term relationships than a single CAHPS score in the clinics or hospitals. Finally, Allina Health is focused on increasingly making the connection between a positive patient experience and the rewards that patient experience will bring for the patient, the physicians and staff, and the organization.

Chapter 13
Case Study: El Camino Hospital

by RJ Salus

El Camino Hospital is a nonprofit organization with hospital locations in Mountain View and Los Gatos, California. The organization has served communities located in the South San Francisco Bay Area for over 50 years. El Camino Hospital Mountain View is a 395-bed hospital located in Silicon Valley. El Camino Hospital Los Gatos is a 143-bed hospital with an ED, medical-surgical, and intensive care services.

Historical Context

As an organization, El Camino had a focus on patient experience dating back to the early 2000s when it worked with the Studer Group and implemented many of Studer's principles. Over the years, with changing leadership, the organization's focus on patient experience had shifted a bit. In 2011, Tomi Ryba became the CEO of El Camino and brought with her a vision for change and a passion for improving the experiences of patients and families. As part of that vision, she started to create her leadership team and structure to help support that vision.

Chapter 13

In 2012, El Camino adopted a continuous improvement approach called Patient Centered Transformation (PaCT). This approach recognizes that traditionally, service, quality, and performance improvement have been viewed as important, but somewhat detached, efforts. PaCT is El Camino Hospital's corrective response to this challenge. PaCT is their patient-centric integrated approach to improve quality, service, and efficiency, via one common set of tools (Lean) supported by a culture of continuous improvement.

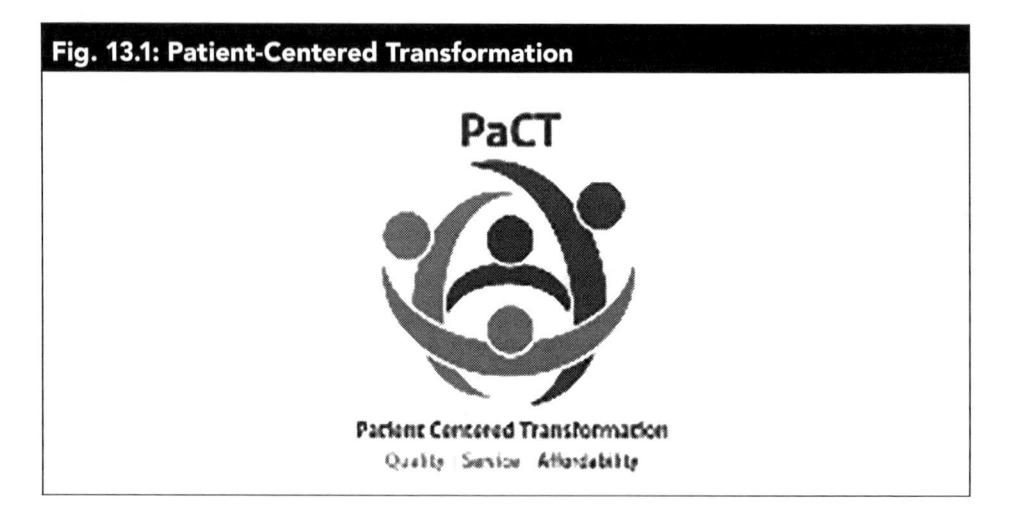

Fig. 13.1: Patient-Centered Transformation

PaCT

Patient Centered Transformation
Quality Service Affordability

El Camino Hospital perceived a gap in its patients' experiences, noted by low HCAHPS scores (bottom quartile in most domains), increased patient complaints, and other quality metrics. The desire was for patients to be surrounded by a culture of service throughout the healing process. Leadership believed this was best achieved by having a personalized approach—created from within their employees' and patients' hearts and minds—an approach that matched the ethos and expectations of the Silicon Valley community. The goal of this work was to achieve top quartile and ultimately top decile patient experience performance through alignment of strategy, measurement, and infrastructure, and by establishing consistency in techniques that solidify standards for service excellence within the organization.

To help them get there, El Camino engaged DTA Associates to facilitate the development of a customized road map using best practices. At El Camino, DTA started with a comprehensive organizational assessment with recommendations tailored to El Camino's current status and future objectives. The outcome was an actionable plan with incremental steps to start implementing right away.

To optimize their internal capacity and to position the organization for success, El Camino leadership aligned their resources to support the improvements. This included creating a director of patient experience role and bringing together some analytical and patient-facing resources. They optimized their existing survey to support measurement of key initiatives and realigned some of their improvement efforts and areas of focus. The creation of a robust PFAC, which consisted of previous patients and/or family members of patients, was essential to this success.

> As we developed our plan to improve the patient experience at our healthcare organization, the voice of the patient was missing. While we knew this was such an important aspect of our journey to improvement, we were not sure where to start.
>
> —Cheryl Reinking, Chief Nursing Officer

To facilitate the creation of performance improvement and training that reflected El Camino's culture as well as the needs of their staff, opportunities were identified through a service-driven culture survey, employee engagement and physician satisfaction surveys, and employee and leadership focus groups. Behavior standards reflecting patients' desires in employees' words were developed and embedded into job descriptions and performance evaluations. Finally, a training plan was developed to determine the content for the various audiences, and tools and videos were created to support skills practice.

Although training offers a wonderful baseline, raises awareness, and propels the culture forward, it often has a "Now what?" phenomenon, in which hospitals fail to maintain momentum and sustain the results. El Camino surmounted this hurdle by retooling, repurposing, and empowering a Patient Experience Committee and by creating a care team coaching program. Care team coaching trained energetic frontline staff role models to shadow other caregivers and provide on-the-spot, nonpunitive feedback.

In addition to the support and structure to improve coupled with the care team coaching for better communication, the other aspects of the El Camino playbook include:

- Performance metrics
  - There was a statistical evaluation on how to prioritize and measure impact that also looked at the key elements of dissatisfaction from a patient perspective, and learned how improvements in those areas would impact overall ratings.
  - Each year there is a review and focus on a few key experience outcome metrics (like nursing communication, medication communication, or staff responsiveness) that align from the organizational level down to the departmental goal. Typically, this also includes some component of process goal as well—for example, a process change with the EMR that will support better pain management for patients.
- Daily huddles
  - Ryba—who led a team to on-site visits at other hospitals that rank best in the country—commented, "One of the better practices we adopted was enterprisewide and department-level daily huddles to support patient safety and service. We review the quality and service experience of patients in a real-time fashion with leaders. At the leader huddle, patient service stories are presented each day, and the progress against our HCAHPS was also tracked as part of the huddle process."

- Voice of the patient

    - El Camino has adopted an approach to performance improvement that weaves in the voice of the patients and families served, sometimes by direct participation of patients in workgroups and committees. The patient voice and storytelling is also integrated into a daily huddle attended by leaders and frontline staff at both facilities. The Patient and Family Advisors provide critical insight and advocacy into initiatives and materials.

    - They also conducted cultural-based patient focus groups. The majority of the moms who deliver babies there are of Chinese and South Asian descent. El Camino is very interested in how to improve their cultural competency and learn the optimal way to support preference and biases, of the mother, partner, husband, and extended family.

- Best practices

    - Implementation of key practices and tracking of those metrics, such as completion of purposeful hourly rounding, use of the care boards, and leadership rounding, have all been part of El Camino's success. Specifically, they have fully adopted multi-disciplinary patient experience rounds which are facilitated by various team members including: environmental services supervisors, nursing leaders, hospital auxilians, the patient experience team, and lab and other ancillary managers. This approach really encourages relationships throughout the continuum of care. A good example of this is the manager of infusion therapy for the outpatient area will round on the oncology unit 4B to see patients while they are still in the hospital. That way she knows them and is a familiar face when they come for their infusion services and outpatient care.

Chapter 13

- Real-time feedback
  - El Camino utilizes multiple platforms to capture real-time feedback, such as a mobile rounding platform to support and track the multidisciplinary rounds, interactive television and media, and a patient hotline.

- Predictive analytics
  - El Camino has utilized an enhanced predictive analytics model to pull from their call light data system as well as their bed alarms in order to help alert management to a potential issue in real time.

- Accountability and incentives
  - At El Camino, functional duties are equally weighted with service behaviors for both employee and leader performance evaluations. Organizational goals are tied to both management and nursing incentive compensation.

- Pre- and posthospital connection
  - El Camino utilizes EMMI, a patient education and engagement platform for patients prior to their surgeries and other procedures. This process was adjusted to enable patients to contact someone prior to their visit. While only used a handful of times, it has been powerful in terms of patient impact and experience.

- Strategic integration
  - At El Camino, each major strategy and even new Information Services requests must articulate their direct and indirect value to patients and families. The recent EPIC implementation included special attention to the use of an EMR as a patient-centered tool.

- Care team coaching
  - El Camino has adopted DTA's nonpunitive and individualized coaching approach to improving patient experience and

communication. The model utilizes six frontline staff, trained to identify key communication practices in action. They shadow other staff (from outside their normal assignment), and it has been a mostly voluntary participation. A few unit partnership councils decided to make it mandatory for their units. To date, 400 staff members have had a coaching experience.

- Patient representatives
  - The complaints and grievance process at El Camino was retooled, and a small team of patient experience representatives who proactively solve problems, create positive experiences, and firefight when necessary, was created to help expedite resolutions to patient concerns.

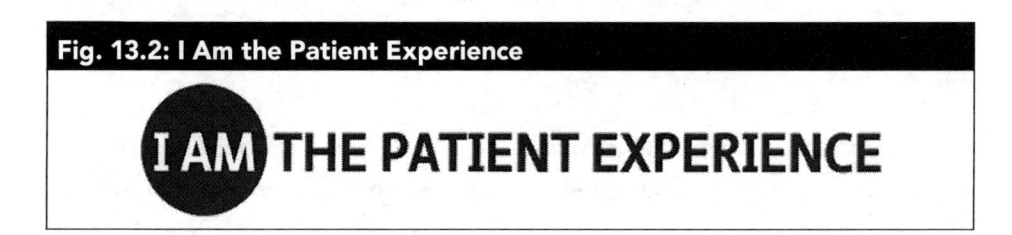

Fig. 13.2: I Am the Patient Experience

I AM THE PATIENT EXPERIENCE

Lessons Learned

Throughout this journey, there have been various lessons learned for El Camino. Some of the biggest include:

- Service culture training is relatively easy to do once you figure out the logistics. Following up with engaged staff members after the training is especially time-consuming and difficult to incorporate consistently. Care team coaching is a great way to reinforce the concepts in the training modules on a personal, individual level.

- Getting frontline staff members' ideas is relatively easy in terms of listening, but keeping them engaged in developing the solution is very challenging. This is due to many issues: budget, staff time allocation to help work on improvements with their work schedules, and staff who don't want to be engaged but would rather just share their idea with someone and let them fix it.

- Physician engagement in a loosely integrated medical staff environment is tough. There are lots of partners and groups to keep up with, and it can be overwhelming to talk to all of them. Additionally, in that type of an environment, it's a balance to help multiple connections and not be seen as playing favorites with one group or organization over another. One of the phenomenal things that helped to change the conversation and these relationships was inviting physicians to the PFAC to hear from the patients firsthand.

- Focusing on service lines as a way to generate engagement and remove barriers is a great way to involve both physicians and frontline staff at the same time. Multidisciplinary groups continue to have more success than working with just one group of caregivers.

- From a performance improvement lens, the A3 format for improvement seems to provide a level of structure for groups that is helpful. Engaging people with a visual management system is also very helpful.

- From a leadership perspective, having an executive who gets it and is passionate is a huge win for the organization. Additionally, having a pragmatist who helps figure out the practical ways to realize and focus the vision is also helpful.

- Midlevel/middle management turnover creates a lot of challenges in getting traction to help keep the patient experience work moving. While it is a challenge, it can also be a success when relationships

Case Study: El Camino Hospital

with those leaders can be developed and they can be equipped with the tools and resources to help connect the dots with their staff.

- An EMR implementation is very distracting and consumes the entire organization. It can take a while to get back to the focus on patient experience even after go-live.

- Recruiting patient advisors to go beyond a monthly meeting format commitment and to get them engaged in performance improvement activities is difficult. This requires some administrative muscle to really keep on these recruitment efforts.

Results: We also have instituted Vis Boards in more than 30 departments that highlight goals in the triple aim: quality, service, and affordability. This is a visual reminder to staff on the key areas of focus.

Our nursing union also adopted as part of the labor contract a special incentive for improved results in service.

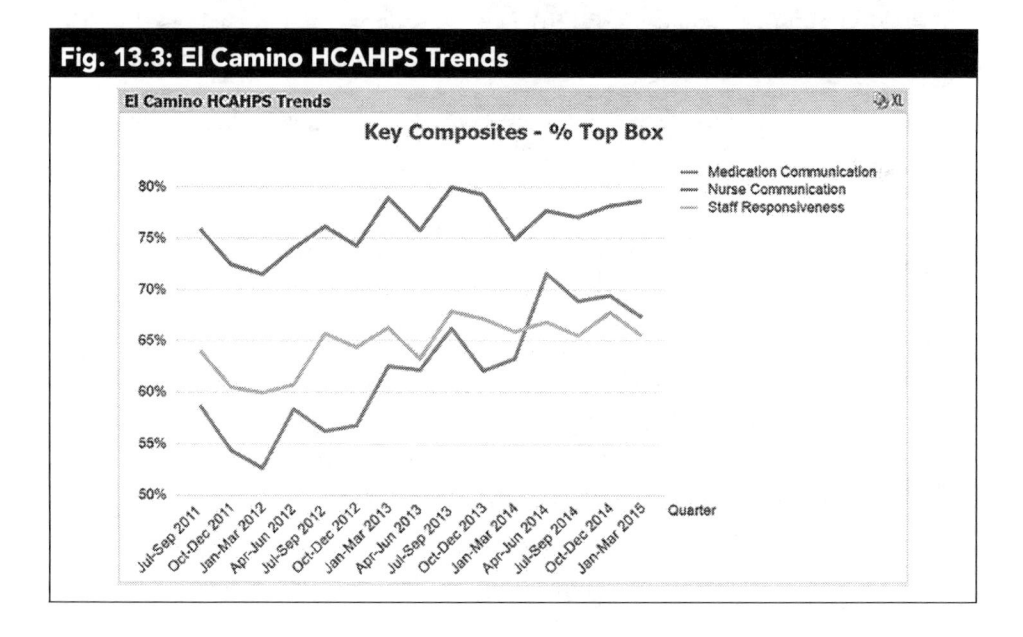

Fig. 13.3: El Camino HCAHPS Trends

Chapter 13

El Camino has seen increases in almost every HCAHPS domain. There has been consistent top-quartile performance in likelihood to recommend and other key metrics.

What's Next?

The work in patient experience and realizing patient- and family-centered care is never done. El Camino continues to move forward in working to further realize their vision. Some of the specific things they are focused on now include:

- Further ensure that the voice of the patient helps to inform the process changes being made in their Lean and performance improvement work.

- Gain back what momentum and traction in improvements and outcomes were lost with the pause for the EMR implementation.

- Expand the focus to work the front-end departments such as the ED and other outpatient areas to get a broader focus to these efforts.

- Enhance the toolkits to support managers as they lead this work on each of their units.

Planetree has been engaged to conduct a gap assessment from the vantage point of patient- and family-centeredness and to help define patient- and family-centered care to every level of the organization.

> Our collective hope is that we are distinguished in our communities by having a patient-centered experience for patients and families. This requires that our culture honors individual preferences and values education, resulting in optimal clinical outcomes and allowing patients to restore their overall health and well-being.
>
> —Tomi Ryba, President and CEO

Chapter 14
Conclusion

We started this journey with an in-depth look at the compulsories of patient experience and examined various means of establishing and sustaining connection with the care team members. We looked at how projecting the voices of patients and families and also focusing on employee engagement are necessary and ongoing processes to ultimately realize the collaboration desired within the organization as well as beyond it. I'm thankful for the way Kevin Campbell illustrated that data is not the ending point but an essential agent in all three of these phases: from understanding the compulsories to how to use data to engage physicians in particular, and ultimately focusing and measuring the collaborative elements for improvement. From there we looked at strategies for how to set the organization up for success both in structure as well as some key aspects of communication. Recognizing that there is no silver bullet, we examined one of the best strategies to help accelerate performance: shadow coaching. I'm grateful to Steve Bergeson, Janet Wied, Tracy Laibson, and RJ Salus for sharing their stories from Allina Health and El Camino Hospital as beautiful illustrations of the concepts shared throughout this book. What I love about their stories is that they're not done. Each of them have work they still want to do to help their organizations realize true patient- and family-centered care.

I mentioned before that when hiring people to work in this area, I looked for those who understood that there was no greater honor than if we worked ourselves out of a job. That means some combination of the following:

- The organization's goals are met: "We hit the coveted 90th+ percentile" or "_____."

- The ownership of this work is so systemically embedded in the leaders of the various sites/units/departments such that everyone sees it as their role.

Today, in my role as a consultant, I see the very same thing. Our approach with the organizations that we work with is that of partnership to help realize their goals and build internal capacity so they are no longer in need of our services.

The reality is that just as for Steve, Janet, Tracy, and RJ, the work in many organizations is not yet done. I find that for many organizations, this is an ongoing journey of continuing connection and collaboration. Many are getting closer and are further along than they were five to seven years ago. My hope is that this guide will help you in your journey, and I hope to hear from you as you progress on it.